OPHTHALMIC ANAESTHESIA

OPHTHALMIC ANAESTHESIA

EDITORS

DR CHANDRA M KUMAR
James Cook University Hospital
Middlesbrough
UK

PROFESSOR CHRIS DODDS
James Cook University Hospital
Middlesbrough
UK

DR GARY L FANNING
Hauser-Ross Eye Institute
Sycamore, Illinois, USA

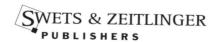

SWETS & ZEITLINGER
PUBLISHERS

LISSE   ABINGDON   EXTON (PA)   TOKYO

Library of Congress Cataloging-in-Publication Data

Applied for

Cover design: Studio Jan De Boer, Amsterdam
Typesetting: Red Barn Publishing, Skeagh, Skibbereen, Co. Cork, Ireland
Printed in the Netherlands by Krips The Print Force, Meppel

Published by: A.A. Balkema Publishers, a member of Swets & Zeitlinger Publishers
www.balkema.nl and www.szp.swets.nl

ISBN 90 265 1928 1

Contents

Preface

Ophthalmic anaesthesia is important for both anaesthetists and ophthalmologists. This book has been written to provide them with the basic knowledge of anatomy, the principles relating to the safe conduct of general and regional anaesthesia in children and adult patients, the specific anaesthetic techniques, and the changes that have occurred in ophthalmic anaesthesia over the last decades. This book will bring together internationally known and respected clinicians from the United Kingdom, Europe, and the USA who have influenced the field of ophthalmic anaesthesia. They have contributed significantly in the field as editors, writing editorials for journals, reviewing articles for journals, and authoring chapters in text books. Many of them have been teaching and demonstrating the techniques of regional anaesthesia for surgery of the eye to their colleagues, endeavouring to make ophthalmic anaesthesia a safer speciality. This book will be of interest to ophthalmologists, ophthalmic anaesthetists and anaesthetic nurses all over the world.

Contributors

Prof Chris Dodds, MBBS, FRCA, MRCGP
Consultant Anaesthetist
James Cook University Hospital
Marton Road
Middlesbrough
TS4 3BW, UK

Mr Timothy C Dowd, FRCOph
North Riding Infirmary
Newport Road
Middlesbrough, UK

Prof Jonathan J Dutton, MD, PhD
Atlantic Eye and Face Center
2501 Western Parkway
Cary
NC 27513, USA

Dr Gary Fanning, MD
Hauser-Ross Eye Institute
2240 Gateway Drive
Sycamore
IL 60178, USA

Dr Marc Feldman, MD, MHS
Cleveland Clinic Foundation Eye Inst
9500 Euclid Avenue
Cleveland
OH 44195, USA

Dr Richard A Fichman, MD
4 Mohawk Dr
West Hartford
CT 06117, USA

Dr Steven Gayer, MD, MBA
Univ of Miami School of Medicine
900 N W 17th St O.R.
Miami
FL 33136, USA

Dr Robert C (Roy) Hamilton, MBBch, FFARCS, FRCP
University of Calgary
University Drive
Calgary AB
T2N 4A9, Canada

Mr Jerry Hill, CRNA
Eye Centers of Florida
Fort Myers
Florida
33901, USA

Dr Robert F Hustead, MD, DABA
4714 N. Portwest Ct
Wichita
KS 67204, USA

Dr Robert W Johnson, MBBS, FRCA
Consultant Anaesthetist
Bristol Royal Infirmary
Bristol, UK

Dr Chandra M Kumar, MBBS, DA, FFARCSI, FRCA, MSc
Consultant Anaesthetist
James Cook University Hospital
Marton Road
Middlesbrough
TS4 3BW, UK

Dr Hamish McLure, FRCA
Consultant Anaesthetist
St James University Hospital
Becket Street
Leeds, UK

Mr B B Patil, FRCS
Department of Ophthalmology
North Riding Infirmary
Newport Road
Middlesbrough, UK

Miss Gina Stancel, RN
Eye Centers of Florida
Fort Myers
Florida
33901, USA

Foreword

The past two decades have seen the publication of eight English language texts devoted solely to ophthalmic anaesthesia.[1–8] The editors of this book have assembled an international group of experts as its authors. Many are members of the Ophthalmic Anesthesia Society (OAS) and the British Ophthalmic Anaesthesia Society (BOAS). The publication is a tribute to the high degree of cooperation existing between these societies from opposite sides of the Atlantic. It is fitting that the opening chapter is a review of the history of ophthalmic anaesthesia authored by the founding presidents of these organisations – Dr Robert Hustead and Dr Robert Johnson respectively.

Most of the readers are expected to be anaesthesiologists. The days are gone when ocular regional anaesthesia was the exclusive domain of the ophthalmic surgeon. Anaesthesiologists have participated in an evolution to establish their role in leading the way to safer practice and more efficient use of operating theatre time.

In this text are the resources of book knowledge in the appropriate basic sciences and clinical skills. For trainees in regional anaesthesia, whether ophthalmic surgeons or anaesthesiologists, observation of and supervision by experienced personnel are essential to complement book knowledge. The goal for each practitioner is to build an experiential database.

In covering newer techniques this book is most timely. Sub-Tenon's and topical corneo-conjunctival anaesthesia are being increasingly used, and yet the tried and true older regional techniques still have their place. All are appropriately described.

Sound anaesthesia principles are the basis for success in all types of surgery. Dependable anaesthesia guidelines are here presented for a range of ophthalmic surgery procedures in adults and children. Readers will find a firm foundation on which to illuminate and build their practices. The closing chapter by Professor Chris Dodds casts an eye to the future.

Dr Robert C (Roy) Hamilton, MBBch, FFARCSI, FRCPC
The University of Calgary Health Sciences Centre
3330 Hospital Drive, NW
Calgary, Alberta
Canada, T2N 4N1

References

1   Bruce RA, McGoldrick KE, Oppenheimer P, eds. *Anesthesia for ophthalmology.* Aesculapius Publishing Company, Birmingham, AL, USA, 1982.
2   Smith GB, ed. *Ophthalmic anaesthesia.* Edward Arnold, London, UK, 1983.

3   Zahl K, Meltzer MA, eds. *Regional anesthesia for intraocular surgery.* Ophthalmology Clinics of North America, Vol. 3, Nr. 1. WB Saunders Company, Philadelphia, PA, USA, 1990.

4   Gills JP, Hustead RF, Sanders DR, eds. *Ophthamic anesthesia.* Slack Incorporated, Thorofare, NJ, USA, 1993.

5   Johnson RW, Forrest FC, eds. *Local and general anaesthesia for ophthalmic surgery.* Butterworth-Heinemann Limited, London, UK, 1994.

6   Smith GB, Hamilton RC, Carr CA, eds. *Ophthalmic anaesthesia.* 2nd ed. Arnold, London, UK, 1996.

7   Greenbaum S, ed. *Ocular anesthesia.* WB Saunders Company, Philadelphia, PA, USA, 1997.

8   Davis DB, Mandel MR, eds. *Anesthesia.* Ophthalmology Clinics of North America, Vol. 11, Nr. 1. WB Saunders Company, Philadelphia, PA, USA, 1998.

1

The History of Ophthalmic Anaesthesia: Clinical Perspectives

Dr Robert F. Hustead
Dr Robert W. Johnson

Introduction

The aim of anaesthesia is to provide excellent conditions for the patient and surgeon taking account of safety, efficacy and efficiency. Not only have there been advances in anaesthesia but also enormous changes in the scope and techniques of surgery. Advances in anaesthesia have both followed surgical technical advances and have permitted them. The rate of change in different parts of the world has varied for many reasons; for instance, in the UK the ready availability of medical specialists in anaesthesia, combined with a slower transition to day-care surgery, delayed the move to local anaesthesia (LA) in ophthalmic surgery.

The development of better drugs of shorter duration of action and reduced toxicity has made general anaesthesia (GA) for ambulatory surgery safer and more common. Advances in the management of the airway, firstly development of the endotracheal tube, intermittent positive pressure ventilation and, more recently, the laryngeal mask airway have allowed avoidance of the operating field and more physiological conditions within the eye during surgery. Similar advances in monitoring have further added to safety.

Local anaesthesia has evolved from simple topical anaesthesia to a broad range of orbital injection techniques. Injection techniques improved with a better understanding of orbital anatomy, the emergence of safer local anaesthetic drugs, and the availability of disposable, purpose-built cannulae and needles.

Ageing of the population is increasing the demands for cataract surgery and expectations for a safe, pain-free and convenient experience. High volume surgical practices have emerged to meet these demands, which will no doubt lead to further advances in anaesthesia and surgical techniques.

The development of general anaesthesia in ophthalmic surgery occurred before local anaesthesia. Each area has shown independent progress and only occasionally have developments in one area directly influenced the other. We summarise highlights of both techniques and relate them to the safety of patients and their visual outcome.

General Anaesthesia

General anaesthesia was introduced in 1846 and became popular with patients because it was such an improvement over restraints, alcohol, opium, or Mesmeric trance. However, the ophthalmologist did not welcome GA because orbital congestion[1] made the operation more difficult and added to the duration of surgery.[2] In addition, the physical proximity of the anaesthetist, trying to keep the patient breathing and alive, led to friction.[1–3] Besides, patients died from anaesthesia. From 1846 to 1884 many of the world's ophthalmologists would operate with the patient in restraints, rather than heed their patient's requests for pain relief. After this time, better techniques for maintaining the airway were gradually introduced, but the introduction of improved general anaesthetic agents did not follow for some time. Improvements in GA for eye surgery were slowed greatly by the introduction of cocaine, the first effective topical anaesthetic. The change from GA to LA was more rapid in the USA; this may have been because there were more trained physician anaesthetists in Europe.

Local Anaesthesia

Koller's pioneering demonstration in 1884[1,4,5] of the anaesthetic effect of topical cocaine to abolish the pain for ophthalmic surgery was a major advance. An early criticism of cocaine was that it caused hazing and damage to the cornea. This concern was addressed by a study of Koller in 1901, reported by Allen[6], in which he repeatedly instilled cocaine into one eye of rabbits, and kept that eye closed. The other eye was simply kept open. Hazing only occurred in the open eye. Enthusiasm quickly returned for topical anaesthesia, with the admonition that the anaesthetized eye should be bathed in its own tears as much as possible until all sensation returned. This study is just as valid today.

Allen[6] also suggested using dilute cocaine to precede strong cocaine to prevent most of the burning and stinging, especially important in the traumatized eye. The topical application of cocaine was only effective for brief, superficial surgery but not for deeper operations. Topical cocaine did not diffuse deeply enough to totally abolish sensation from the iris in most patients and did not abolish pain of the pull on muscles or the cutting of the optic nerve[1,6] even when placed next to the globe through incisions in the bulbar conjunctiva by Turnbull.[7]

In 1884, Knapp[1] succeeded in making the patient more comfortable during deeper operations in the eye with multiple injections of cocaine — under the conjunctiva, around the muscles and optic nerve — and many ophthalmologists adopted this. Despite sedatives and morphine, many patients continued to have pain and would squint their eyes, making it difficult for the surgeon to complete the operation. It became possible to prevent patients from squinting or closing their eyes with the addition of orbicularis akinesia by a facial nerve block that was introduced by Van Lint in 1914[8] and improved upon by Wright[9] and O'Brien.[10] However, as a result of pain, many would still strain and move about, compromising the surgical field. Heavy sedation controlled this activity and was often started the day before surgery and continued through the prolonged convalescence.[10] This was the state of anaesthesia for the majority of patients having cataract surgery through the 1930s.

Topical cocaine was gradually replaced by tetracaine 1% in the 1930s, even though the replacement drugs did not dilate the pupil nor provide the vasoconstriction of cocaine. Later replacements included proparacaine in the 1960s and then lidocaine and bupivacaine in the 1990s. Unlike cocaine, the safety of the newer topical anaesthetics has been tested in both animal and in vitro studies, and in randomised clinical trials. Topical anaesthesia for cataract surgery was gradually abandoned after the late 1930s and did not reappear significantly for cataract surgery until the last decade.

Injection of cocaine into the orbit was the logical extension of a purely topical approach enabling the surgeon to reduce the pain from the deeper structures and to provide akinesia of the globe. Knapp[1] reported such injections within weeks of the report of Koller's discovery of the topical effectiveness of cocaine and within days after seeing that topical, subconjunctival, and subcutaneous injections were inadequate to block deeper pain. Conduction anaesthesia within the orbit was established with Knapp's documentation of many successes and with the subsequent reports of Lowenstein[3] and Allen.[6] Cocaine caused relatively little pain on injection, produced excellent vasoconstriction, and blocked sensory and motor nerves.

However, LA injection in the orbit was slow to gain acceptance because large volume orbital injection often caused pain and side effects such as syncope, cold sweats, and hallucinations, which were rare with topical administration of cocaine. Some patients still experienced pain during surgery despite the orbital injections. In the first published reports of cocaine injection for enucleation in the United States, Knapp reported syncope with 0.37 ml (6 minims) of 2% cocaine. Knapp described forced traction on the globe following which the patient undoubtedly experienced a vasovagal syncope. Knapp interpreted this reaction as 'toxicity of cocaine in the vascular orbit,' and warned of the possibility of death had a larger amount of cocaine been used[1] urging that even smaller volumes of cocaine be used henceforth.

The concept of using minimal volumes of cocaine in the orbit was established because of Knapp's observations and reports. His failure to differentiate systemic or local toxicity from the vasomotor effects of painful injection, muscle traction and pain from non-anaesthetized areas established a false basis for regional anaesthesia in the orbit that was hard to overcome. Orbital injection techniques only gradually became accepted because of: (1) reports of reactions when cocaine was injected around or behind the eye, (2) the cost of having the sterile injectable reliable cocaine solution prepared on a daily basis, (3) reports of blindness and death from intra-orbital injection of cocaine, and (4) reports of injections being ineffective in the relief of deep orbital pain. Injection deep enough or in adequate amount to block the ciliary ganglion was reserved for enucleation[11,12] because of the fear of producing blindness in a sighted eye by intraorbital injections.

Because of the morbidity and poor operating conditions under general anaesthesia Elschnig and Lowenstein[3] persisted in trying to achieve anaesthesia with LA for enucleation and other deep eye surgery. They were able to accomplish painless enucleation in 98% of patients using nerve block with cocaine and epinephrine. Lowenstein injected cocaine in the area of the ciliary ganglion with spread of anaesthetic to the optic nerve sheath, the nearby oculomotor and naso-ciliary nerves, and separately to the sensory nerves to the conjunctiva, proving that a total block could be done with less than half the accepted toxic dose of cocaine.[3]

The observation of calmness and freedom from pain in patients having enucleation led Duverger[2] to use the Prague method also. Impressed with its effectiveness, he started using local anaesthetic injections in the area of the ciliary ganglion for patients in whom he expected difficulty during cataract surgery. Blockade of the ciliary ganglion, ciliary nerves, the naso-ciliary nerve, and the sensory nerves to the lids and conjunctiva, led to freedom of pain from cataract surgery and better control of the eye. Direct block of the facial nerve was a useful adjunct to prevent inadvertent eye closure and to decrease the pressure of the muscles on the globe.

Thus by the 1920s, Lowenstein and Duverger had established that excellent surgical conditions for cataract surgery as well as enucleation could be safely provided by regional orbital block, which they called 'ciliary ganglion block', although many other nerves were blocked in addition. Gifford[13] in the US recognised that those who had adopted 'ciliary ganglion block' had a much higher frequency of excellent surgical results.[2,14,15]

The major proponent of ciliary ganglion block, facial block, and globe paresis for cataract surgery in the United States was Atkinson, who reported his technique and its benefits every 3–5 years.[16–23] Atkinson's intraconal ciliary ganglion block became known as the 'retrobulbar block.' The success of the intraconal block led to the explosion of regional anaesthesia for cataract surgery of the 1940s and 50s. At this time the majority of these blocks were performed by the surgeon (in the USA), with general anaesthesia remaining the predominant method in many other parts of the world.

Some patients still had pain and would strain at the wrong time from inadequate single-needle injection of 'retrobulbar' anaesthesia, and some patients would not develop akinesia, which led some US surgeons to adopt GA, administered by anaesthesiologists or nurse anaesthetists, and others to adopt the apical injection of Gifford.[13,24] Many surgeons, as recommended by Atkinson, just added more LA to their 'retrobulbar blocks' and made intraorbital injections of the sensory nerves. Such techniques allowed painless enucleation, re-establishing that injections of LA were effective as reported by Lowenstein in 1908 and Duverger in 1920.

Atkinson referred to Knapp's technique as the first retrobulbar nerve block.[21,23] Knapp referred to his own technique as an injection close to the posterior surface of the globe to block the ciliary nerves. Atkinson refers to this first retrobulbar block as producing retrobulbar anaesthesia for painless enucleation. The block was retrobulbar in anatomical terms, but was not an Atkinson retrobulbar block, and it did not produce anaesthesia for painless enucleation. The block done by Knapp was much closer to the superonasal injection described by Kirby[25] than it was to an Atkinson block. Confusion over nomenclature persists to this day and a universally accepted taxonomy is much needed

Local Anaesthetic Agents and Adjuvants

Because cocaine worked even better when epinephrine was added, the search for an 'ideal' ophthalmic LA gained little momentum. Epinephrine was found to extend useful anaesthesia time with cocaine, decrease vitreous pressure, decrease bleeding, and decrease the amount of local anaesthetic needed. Most eye surgery did not require dangerously large amounts of cocaine, and it provided better conditions than other drugs available at the time.

Procaine

In general surgery procaine replaced cocaine after 1902 because it was safer. Procaine became more useful when epinephrine was added to obtain vasoconstriction and satisfactory anaesthesia but only gradually replaced cocaine in ophthalmology because of cocaine's familiarity. O'Brien, in 1928, recommended 0.3 ml of cocaine 4% mixed equally with 1:1,000 epinephrine at the 12 o'clock conjunctival position to anaesthetize the conjunctiva and iris.[10]

Procaine eventually became the standard local anaesthetic agent for injection in ophthalmology. It was non-addictive, was more stable in solution, had a longer shelf life, and could be purchased in bottles ready for use. Cocaine had to be prepared almost daily by the pharmacist to be reliable, and drug laws required strict record keeping. The concept of injection of minimal amounts of LA for eye surgery, based upon the early clinical observations of cocaine and procaine/epinephrine mixtures, delayed the more rational use of procaine and the other LA drugs that followed.

Minimal doses of procaine were injected in the orbit, as with cocaine, because of fear of sudden death from injection and because larger injections were known to elevate intraorbital volume and intraocular pressure (IOP). Procaine was rapidly removed from the orbit and the block fleeting unless it was combined with high dose epinephrine. The added epinephrine was shown to decrease IOP and was therefore added in amounts of 1:1,000 to 1:5,000 by those promoting injection technique. Many patients exhibited toxic reaction to the procaine/epinephrine combination when this was injected in the orbit in any but the smallest quantity. Larger quantities could cause syncope and cold sweats similar to that reported with cocaine.

Hyaluronidase

Techniques using small amounts of procaine and large amounts of sedation would have remained the techniques of choice for cataract surgery until today, if not for Atkinson's report in 1949 that larger doses of LA to produce akinesia could be injected in the cone if hyaluronidase was injected along with it and if the globe was massaged to get rid of the excess fluid. His recommended dose of 2% procaine in the muscle cone for cataract surgery went up from 1 ml in 1934[16] to 1–1.5 ml in 1949[19] after the addition of hyaluronidase, and even higher in subsequent years.

The reliability, safety, and effectiveness of the larger dose of procaine/hyaluronidase mixture for retrobulbar injection was becoming a well-accepted practice when it was noted that hyaluronidase could be added to lidocaine solution, which had recently been introduced into the American market.[26] The volume of the newer, safer anaesthetic, lidocaine, could be increased considerably without causing more than a temporary increase in IOP, which could be eliminated by massaging the globe to spread the anaesthetic and facilitate absorption.

Atkinson encouraged the use of lidocaine because it was safer and spread better than procaine[20–23] and recommended injection into the safer intraconal compartment. The recommended volume of local increased to the amount producing noticeable proptosis, 2–3 ml in 1955[20] and 4 ml or more up to 8 ml in 1964.[22] He conservatively recommended in the second edition of his book[23] in 1965, a volume of '3 ml or more in the average orbit and more being frequently useful.' The combination of hyaluronidase, larger anaesthetic volume, and prolonged, deliberate pressure over the orbit was shown by Kirsch[27] to produce the hypotony of the globe desired for ideal intracapsular cataract extraction. This hypotony by ocular compression with reduction of vitreous volume produced conditions that would allow time and space to do the operation expeditiously, despite the early worry that too soft an eye created problems in lens extraction. The soft eye and vitreous dehydration allowed space for lens prosthesis implantation, which was to follow in a few years.

Newer LA Drugs

Lidocaine was recommended even though it seemed to be more painful on injection.[22,23,26,28] However, lidocaine did not seem to last long enough when the time-consuming extracapsular surgery with lens implantation was introduced. Hence, the longer-lasting LA mepivacaine[29] gained some proponents whilst others added tetracaine[25,30] to lidocaine, bupivacaine to lidocaine[31] or bupivacaine alone.[31] Etidocaine[32] which worked as fast as lidocaine and lasted as long as bupivacaine, was not accepted in ophthalmology because of pain on injection and reports of prolonged muscle paresis.

These drugs or combinations caused much more pain on injection than did procaine, but they proved longer lasting. The longer-acting bupivacaine appeared to have less spreading effect and much slower onset than lidocaine, and volumes of 5 ml or more of a lidocaine/bupivacaine mixture were becoming standard in much the same way that large volumes of lidocaine had been encouraged by Atkinson.[23] The mixture of lidocaine/bupivacaine provided longer blocks and postoperative analgesia, which patients appreciated. This would allow regional anaesthesia to become useful for longer procedures such as scleral buckle and vitrectomy.

The search for an ideal LA seemed to be satisfied by lidocaine/bupivacaine or mepivacaine/bupivacaine mixtures despite textbook authors suggesting that mixtures had no logical place.[33] However, incomplete akinesia of the extraocular muscles was not rare with the new mixtures. The variability of obtaining ocular akinesia had always been an inconvenience, but the impression that vitreous loss was caused by a moving eye was becoming established. This could now be solved with the addition of bupivacaine or etidocaine to the armamentarium, by increasing the volume of injectate, and then ocular compression to reduce orbital volume and IOP.

Other Considerations

Blocking outside the operating room was a totally new concept in many private hospitals in the US and was not encouraged by many hospitals. It was always considered mandatory for the surgeons to block their own patients in the operating room. The block and the ten minutes of digital ocular massage were considered part of operating room procedure and efficiency was ignored.

Improvements in drugs and techniques allowed greater efficiency leading to greater throughput. Ambulatory surgery centres with dedicated anaesthesia personnel emerged, and high-volume cataract surgery subsequently increased worldwide. It is salutary that Indian eye camps have provided such surgery for several decades to the benefit of many.

The move to outpatient surgery discouraged sedation. It had long been questioned whether sedatives increased the safety of the relatively small amounts of LA used in ophthalmic surgery. Long-lasting oral or intramuscular sedatives interfered with early ambulation and required additional attendants. Some patients benefited from the short, rapid-acting sedatives given prior to the block because that was the only painful part of the entire procedure. It was then realised that the block could be made even less painful by eliminating the orbicularis block[34] which had become unnecessary with large-volume orbital injections and by using painless or almost painless topical anaesthetics prior to transconjunctival retrobulbar block[34] and painless injectable LA[35] with slow injection of body temperature anaesthetic solutions.[36] Using such techniques, sedation could be reduced or eliminated for most patients. It was also noted that it was becoming easier to diagnose the difference between poor and good blocks, as the patients were very alert when they had no sedative. Akinesia and anaesthesia could be assessed before the patient went to the operating room with great assurance of a pain-free experience.

The danger of injection deep into the orbital apex had been known for 100 years as a cause of blindness and death. This was known to those who used: (1) the inferotemporal approach, viz., Lowenstein,[3] Duverger,[2] Allen,[6] Labat,[37] Atkinson,[16,23]

Gifford[24] (2) the superotemporal route, viz., Knapp,[1] Braun,[38] Pitkin[39] and (3) the superonasal route, viz., Peuckart.[6] Most authors tried to prevent these disasters by applying knowledge of orbital anatomy, but Atkinson and Gifford additionally extolled the use of specially prepared dull needles. Even though the optic nerve and central artery could not be perforated with such dull needles in dogs in the laboratory, human cases still occurred with dull needles. A combination of circumstances brought with it reports of patients who would stop breathing from two to ten minutes after the injection of anaesthetic. Whereas direct injection into the subarachnoid space by the needle was by far the best explanation, the possibility of epidural spread was never eliminated. No deaths were reported in over 50 of these episodes because of the timely intervention of anaesthesia providers. As a result, the use of anaesthesia personnel in the ophthalmic surgery theatre became logical both to block and monitor the patients, provided they were trained in ophthalmic local anaesthesia. The Guidelines for LA for cataract surgery published in 1993 jointly by the Royal College of Anaesthetists and the College of Ophthalmologists, whilst far from perfect, raised awareness of the risks of LA and their avoidance.

Brainstem anaesthesia was at first blamed on bupivacaine until it was established that it could occur with lidocaine/bupivacaine mixtures or lidocaine alone and that it was more frequent with large volume injections, longer and sharper needles, and intraconal or apical block techniques. The potential pathway was then demonstrated for anaesthetic to enter the mid-brain via the orbital extension of the subarachnoid covering of the optic nerve sheath.[40] Dynamic CT scans by Unsold[41] showed the optic nerve and central retinal artery moved about in the orbit and could be placed in the pathways of needles during movement of the eye when asking the patient to 'look up and in' as recommended by Atkinson. Furthermore, the globe could be seen rotating its posterior pole in the direction opposite to the anterior hemisphere when digital pressure was applied to elevate the anterior globe. Thus the optic nerve is placed at more risk of injury than Atkinson and those before had taught.

Katsev[42] measured the orbits of many humans and showed that orbital lengths vary considerably. Their work demonstrated that the commonly used 1½" needle could reach dangerous areas of the orbital apex in 15–20% of patients, regardless of the approach of the orbital block.

Techniques were described in the 1980s to eliminate penetration of the optic nerve sheath and needle damage to the optic nerve and the central retinal artery. These were based on the pre-1970s concept of the anatomy of the orbit that considered the orbit to be divided into two compartments: (1) the intraconal space contained by the extraocular muscles and intermuscular septum and (2) the extraconal space or the space between the orbital bones and the intraconal space. Injections to provide anaesthesia for orbital surgery were then described as being safer when placed in the extraconal space by Davis,[43] Bloomberg[44] and Weiss[45] and just as effective as intraconal injections. These safer spaces were called peribulbar by Davis[43] or periocular by Bloomberg or Weiss.[44,45] It was true that the injections intended to go in this space could bring about anaesthesia and akinesia, but how could LA placed outside the muscle cone penetrate inside the muscle cone to block the intraconal nerves to the globe and extraocular muscles?

An anatomist/ophthalmologist, Koornneef[46] made anatomical reconstructions of the human orbit from a large number of specimens of many ages which showed that there was no complete 'intermuscular septum' dividing the orbit into intraconal and extraconal compartments, except near the insertion of the muscles to the globe, or deep in the orbital apex. There were adipose tissue compartments between the muscles through which anaesthetic drugs could move in the orbit and could readily anaesthetize intraconal nerves. Newer techniques using this information were described in the late 1980s and 1990s allowing needles to be placed more safely into the muscle cone with the eye in primary[47,48] or upward gaze[34] without reaching the optic nerve or orbital apex provided that appropriate sites of insertion, correct trajectories, and appropriate needle lengths were used. These techniques did place needles further away from the optic nerve but required larger volumes to be injected for effectiveness than either Atkinson's conal or Gifford's apical techniques.

The volume of injectate recommended for the new techniques varied from 3–10 mL using either a single injection or multiple injections into 'safe areas.' The 'safe areas' described were (1) more anteriorly in the cone than the standard cone injection of Atkinson, and with the eyes straight ahead as described by Gills/Loyd[34] or Hamilton[49] or above the eye as by Kelman[50] and Thornton[51] (2) into the lateral cone as in the block by Gills and Loyd[34] (3) outside the cone in the anterior peribulbar sites of Davis[36], the anterior peribulbar sites of Wang[52] or the periocular sites of Weiss[43] and Bloomberg[53] (4) the medial periconal site of Hustead[54] or (5) sub-Tenon's injection[25] under direct vision or with a cannula as advocated by Greenbaum.[55]

Single injection techniques had their own problems. From 3 to 20% of patients needed a second injection or additional injections in two or more sites to provide complete akinesia. Optimum insertion sites and safer trajectories of needle paths seemed to be key in providing total akinesia and anaesthesia whilst keeping the patient and globe safe. Rare but serious complications continued to be reported.

Much controversy remained as to whether it was safer to put dull needles or sharp needles into the orbit or whether the needle should be straight or curved. Large dull needles can cause more damage to sight and the globe[56] than do fine sharp needles, and the debate continues. The attempts by Straus[57] to use a curved needle with a known radius and short straight segment and Hamilton's custom bent needle[58] would eventually cause injury as had the curved needle of Siegrist before 1900. Again the debate continues regarding the shape of the needle.

Whilst the new anatomically driven incentive to teaching safer needle techniques was growing, there was a significant change in surgical technique for cataract surgery. Extracapsular cataract surgery was changing to small incision phacoemulsification and implantation of small profile lenses. Many surgeons were beginning to feel that the marked hypotony produced by ocular compression was unnecessary for less invasive cataract surgical techniques. In fact, some considered it a hindrance for phacoemulsification. Fichman[59] and Fine[60] reported good results using topical anaesthesia without akinesia during phacoemulsification. Many surgeons avidly encouraged topical anaesthesia and many encouraged sub-Tenon's injection with a blunt cannula.[54] Unfortunately, topical alone is not applicable to all patients needing eye surgery, and the need for safer use of needles or blunt cannulae in the orbit continues.

References

1   Knapp H. On cocaine and its use in ophthalmic and general surgery. *Arch Ophthalmol.* 1884; 13:402.
2   Duverger. *L'anesthésie locale en ophtalmologie.* Masson et Cie, Paris, 1920.
3   Lowenstein A. Ueber regionare anasthesie in der orbita. *Klin Monatsbl Augenheilk.* 1908; 592–601.
4   Koller C(K). The use of anaesthesia LA on the eye. Preliminary report. Translation of Koller's preliminary report of Sept 15, 1884. Presented by Dr Brettaur in: Faulconer A, Keys TE (eds). *Foundations of Anesthesiology.* Charles C. Thomas, Springfield, 1965.
5   Koller K. On the use of cocaine to anaesthetize the eye. As translated by H Knapp in On Cocaine and Its Use in Ophthalmic and General Surgery. *Arch Ophthalmol.* 1884; 13:402–448. Translation of Koller's early pharmacology as reported in Oct 25 and Nov 1, Wein Med Wochenscreib 1884.
6   Allen CW. *Local and regional anaesthesia,* second edition. WB Saunders Company, 1918. p 527–530.
7   Turnbull CS. Editorial. *Med Surg Rep.* 1884; 29:628.
8   Van Lint A. Paralysie palpébrale temporarie provoquée dans l'opération de la cataract. *Ann Ocul (Paris).* 1914; 151:420.
9   Wright RE. Blocking of the main trunk of the facial nerve in surgery. *Arch Ophthalmol.* 1926; 55:55–56.
10   O'Brien CS. Akinesis during cataract extraction. *Arch Ophthalmol.* 1929; 1:447–449.
11   Seidel E. Ueber eine Modifikation der Seigristschen Methode der lokal Anesthesie bei Exenteratio und Enuclatio Bulbi. *Klin Monatsbl Augenheilk.* 1911; 49:329.
12   Siegrist A. Lokalanästhesie bei Exentertio und Enucleatio Bulbi. *Klin Monatsbl Augenheilk.* 1907; 5:106–109.
13   Gifford SR. The prevention of complications in the cataract operation. *Ill Med J.* 1935; 68:243–244.
14   Greenwood A, Grossman HP. Analysis of 1,343 intracapsular cataract extractions by 48 operators following the Verhoett method. *Trans Am Ophthalmol Soc.* 1935; 33:353–361.
15   de Grosz E. L'extraction de la cataract d'après 15,000 opérations. *Arch Ophthalmol* 1936; 53:161–165.
16   Atkinson WS. Anaesthesia LA in ophthalmology. *Trans Am Ophthalmol Soc.* 1934; 32:399–451.
17   Atkinson WS. Anaesthesia LA in ophthalmology. *Arch Ophthalmol.* 1943; 30:777–780.
18   Atkinson WS. Anaesthesia LA in ophthalmology. *Am J Ophthalmol.* 1948; 31:1607–1618.
19   Atkinson WS. Use of hyaluronidase with anaesthesia LA in ophthalmology. *Arch Ophthalmol.* 1949; 42:628–633.
20   Atkinson WS. *Anaesthesia in ophthalmology,* first edition. Charles C. Thomas, Springfield, 1955.
21   Atkinson WS. Ophthalmic anaesthesia: the development of ophthalmic anaesthesia. *Am J Ophthalmol.* 1961; 51:1–14.

22   Atkinson WS. Larger volume retrobulbar injections. *Am J Ophthalmol.* 1964; 57:328.
23   Atkinson WS. *Anaesthesia in ophthalmology*, second edition. Charles C. Thomas, Springfield, 1965.
24   Gifford H Jr. Motor block of extraocular muscles by deep orbital injection. *Arch Ophthalmol.* 1949; 41:5–19.
25   Kirby DB. *Surgery of cataract*. JB Lippincott, Philadelphia, 1950.
26   Russell DA, Guyton JS. Retrobulbar injection of lidocaine (Xylocaine) for anaesthesia and akinesia. *Am J Ophthalmol.* 1954; 38:78–84.
27   Kirsch RE. Further studies on the use of digital pressure in cataract surgery. *Arch Ophthalmol.* 1957; 58:641–644.
28   Wightman MA, Vaughan RW. Comparison of compounds used for intradermal anaesthesia. *Anesthesiology.* 1976; 45:687–689.
29   Laaka V, Nikki P, Tarkkanen A. Comparison of bupivacaine with and without adrenalin and mepivacaine with adrenalin in intraocular surgery. *Acta Ophthalmol.* 1972; 50:229–239.
30   Scheie HG, Ellis RA, et al. Long-lasting LA agents in ophthalmic surgery. *Arch Ophthalmol.* 1955; 53:177–190.
31   Gills JP, Rudisill JE. Bupivacaine in cataract surgery. *Ophthalmic Surgery* 1974; 5:67–70.
32   Gutman H, Sinskey RM, et al. A comparison of lidocaine and etidocaine in retrobulbar anaesthesia for cataract surgery. *J Am Intraocul Implant Soc.* 1979; 5:120–122.
33   Miller RD (ed). *Anaesthesia*, third edition. Churchill Livingstone, New York, 1990. p 453.
34   Gills JP, Loyd TL. A technique of retrobulbar block with paralysis of orbicularis oculi. *J Am Intraocul Implant Soc.* 1983; 9:339–340.
35   Hustead, RF. BSS takes the sting out of LA. *Ocul Surg News.* 1986; 4:39.
36   Davis II DB, Mandel MR. Peribulbar anaesthesia, a review of technique and complications. *Ophthalmol Clinics North America.* 1990; 3:101–109.
37   Adriani J (ed). *Labat's regional anaesthesia: techniques and clinical applications*, fourth edition. Warren H. Green, Inc., St. Louis, 1985.
38   Braun H. *Anaesthesia*. Translated and edited by Harris ML. Lea & Febiger, Philadelphia, 1924. pp 180, 218–219, 239.
39   Pitkin GP. *Conduction anaesthesia*. Ed. Southworth JL, Hingson RA. JB Lippincott Co., Philadelphia, 1946. p 337. Second edition, 1953, p 410.
40   Drysdale DB. Experimental subdural retrobulbar injection of anesthetic. *Ann Ophthalmol.* 1984:16; 717–718.
41   Unsold R, Stanley J, Degroot J. The CT topography of retrobulbar anaesthesia. *A Graef Arch Klin Ophthalmol.* 1981; 217:125–136.
42   Katsev DA, Drews RC, Rose BT. An anatomic study of retrobulbar needle path length. *Ophthalmology.* 1989; 96:1221–1224.
43   Davis DB II, Mandel MR. Posterior peribulbar anaesthesia:An alternative to retrobulbar anaesthesia. *J Cataract Refract Surg.* 1986; 12:182–184.
44   Bloomberg L. Periocular method of anaesthesia administration called safe, easy. *Ophthal Times.* 1986; 54–55.
45   Weiss J, Deichman C. A comparison of retrobulbar and periocular anaesthesia for cataract surgery. *Arch Ophthalmol.* 1989; 107:96–98.
46   Koornneef L. New insights in the human orbital connective tissue. *Arch Ophthalmol.* 1977; 95:1269–1273.
47   Pautler SE, Grizzard WS. Blindness from retrobulbar injection into the optic nerve. *Ophthalmic Surgery* 1986; 17:334–337.
48   Hamilton RC, Gimbel HV, Strunin L. Regional anaesthesia for 12,000 cataract extraction and intraocular lens implantation procedures. *Can J Anaesth.* 1988; 35:615–623.

49   Hustead RF, Hamilton RC. In: Techniques: Gills JP, Hustead RF, Sanders DR, editors. *Ophthalmic anaesthesia*. Slack, Thorofare, NJ, 1993.

50   Kelman C. Forward. In: Greenbaum S, editor. *Ocular anesthesia*. Philadelphia, PA: WB Saunders 1997.

51   Thornton SP Ocular anaesthesia with the Thornton retrobulbar needle. In: Techniques: Gills JP, Hustead RF, Sanders DR, editors. *Ophthalmic anesthesia*. Slack, Thorofare, NJ, 1993.

52   Wang HS. Peribulbar anesthesia for ophthalmic procedures. *J Cataract Refract Surg*. 1998; 14:441.

53   Bloomberg L. Anterior periocular anesthesia. In: Davis DB II, Mandel MR, editors. *Ophthalmol Clinics North America*. 1998; 11:47–56.

54   Hustead RF, Hamilton RC, Loken RG. Periocular local anesthesia: Medial orbital as an alternative to superior nasal injection. *J Cataract Refract Surg*. 1994; 20:197–201.

55   Greenbaum S. Parabulbar anesthesia. *Am J Ophthalmol*. 1992; 114:776.

56   Grizzard WS. Ophthalmic anesthesia. In: Reinecke RD, editor. *Ophthalmology annual*. Raven Press, New York, 1989.

57   Straus JG. A new retrobulbar needle and injection technique. *Ophthalmic Surgery* 1998; 19:134.

58   Hamilton RC. In: Smith, Hamilton, Carr, editors. 2nd edition. *Ophthalmic anaesthesia*. Arnold, London, 1996. pp 104–147.

59   Fichman RA. Topical eye drops replace injection for anesthesia. *Ocul Surg News*. 1992; 10:1.

60   Fine IH, Fichman RA, Grabow HB, editors. *Clear-corneal cataract surgery and topical anesthesia*. Slack, Thorofare, NJ, 1993.

2

Anatomic Considerations in Ophthalmic Anaesthesia

Prof. Jonathan J. Dutton

Introduction

Ophthalmic anaesthesia has evolved over the decades into a sophisticated art, which provides comfort to the patient, allays anxiety, and allows the safe execution of delicate eye surgery. Whilst the retrobulbar block has been a standard for many decades, newer techniques, such as the peribulbar and sub-Tenon's blocks and, more recently, topical anaesthesia have gained in popularity over the past several years. These 'less invasive' techniques have been promoted in order to reduce the risks of complications whilst still achieving satisfactory patient comfort.[1-3] Knowledge of local and regional anatomy is essential in order to achieve the proper levels of sensory and motor blockade with minimal complications, regardless of the specific technique employed.[4]

Anatomically Related Complications

Retrobulbar Block

For the retrobulbar and peribulbar blocks, a clear three-dimensional concept of orbital anatomy is essential to avoid injury to the orbital contents. Potential complications include globe perforation, optic nerve injury, subarachnoid injection, extraocular muscle injury, and orbital haemorrhage, among others. Globe perforation has been reported in as many as 0.75% of retrobulbar and peribulbar injections and has been reported with both sharp and blunt needles.[5-9] Most commonly this involves a tangential penetration in the inferolateral quadrant and may include penetration of the inferior oblique muscle as well. Retinal detachment and vitreous haemorrhage are common sequellae, with potential for visual loss.

Careful observation of the globe during needle entry may alert the surgeon or anaesthetist to impending globe penetration by rotation of the eye toward the direction of needle entry. The so-called 'wiggle test' has been advocated to determine if the needle tip has impaled an orbital structure fixed to the eye. In this test, after the retrobulbar needle is in the orbit, but before any anaesthetic is injected, the needle is moved from side to side; any rotation of the eye suggests that the sclera, optic nerve, or an extraocular muscle may have been penetrated. However, this can only increase the scale of damage if the eye has been penetrated (see Chapter 14).

Injection of local anaesthetic into the eye is a potentially devastating complication. The sclera is only 0.8 to 1.0 mm in thickness and offers little resistance to perforation by a needle. Because the injection is into a closed space, resistance to fluid injection is elevated and should therefore alert the operator to this event. Application of very little pressure at the plunger head of the syringe can translate into more than 3000 mm Hg of intraocular pressure, enough to rupture the globe.[10] Larger syringes have less mechanical advantage and, therefore, markedly reduce the risk.

Injection of anaesthetic directly into the optic nerve can result in severe injury and immediate blindness. The injection pressure will be high, which should alert the operator of impending disaster. It is equally important to avoid penetration of the optic nerve sheath and injection of anaesthetic into the subarachnoid space. This compartment contains cerebrospinal fluid in communication with the subdural intracranial and spinal CSF. Injection of anaesthetic into this space may result in sensory blockade of contralateral vision, CNS depression, paralysis, seizures, hypotension, cardiac arrest, and even death.[11-16]

Injury to an extraocular muscle may be missed, since there is very little resistance to needle penetration. The muscles most likely to be injured during needle entry are the inferior oblique or the inferior rectus muscles. Whilst the inferior oblique does not contain ciliary vessels, it is a large and thick muscle that is highly vascular, and its location along the inferolateral globe back to the macula makes it particularly vulnerable to retrobulbar needle entry.

Some concentrated local anaesthetics are toxic to striated muscle tissue. Inadvertent injection can result in muscle dysfunction ranging from mild and temporary paralysis to marked fibrosis.[17] Postoperative muscle dysfunction may be seen even without any clinical evidence of muscle penetration and is the most frequent cause of postoperative strabismus following cataract or scleral bucking procedures.[18-21] In rare instances the strabismus may be neuropathic due to injury to a cranial nerve near the orbital apex.

The anterior ciliary arteries originate in the posterior orbit from the ophthalmic artery and penetrate the posterior one third of the rectus muscles on the conal surface. These vessels run anteriorly and centrally within the muscle bellies and then on the outer surface of the muscle tendons to their points of insertion on the globe. These vessels then penetrate the sclera through emissary canals to supply the ciliary body, iris, and anterior choroidal circulation. The anterior ciliary vessels may be injured by the retrobulbar needle, resulting in retrobulbar haemorrhage or bleeding directly into an extraocular muscle.

Orbital haemorrhage is the most common complication of retrobulbar injection, reported in 0.1% to 1.7% of procedures.[12,22,23] The orbit is highly vascular and contains numerous arteries and veins, as well as the ciliary vessels within the extraocular muscles. Most of the larger vessels are located in the superior and medial orbit making these regions more vulnerable to vascular injury. The quadrant most devoid of larger vascular elements is inferolateral, and this is true of both the intraconal and extraconal compartments. Subperiosteal haemorrhage can occur from contact of the needle with the orbital floor, and in one case this resulted in blindness.[24] Whilst most orbital hemorrhagic events resolve uneventfully, an acute bleed can be localised within an orbital septal fascial system producing a compartment syndrome. The resulting optic nerve and superior ophthalmic vein compression may cause visual loss or an excessive rise in intraocular pressure.

Retrobulbar injection can also significantly reduce pulsatile ocular blood flow by about 250 μl/minute.[25] This might have the potential to alter intraocular pressure, and could compromise eyes with borderline blood flow.

Sub-Tenon's Block
In the sub-Tenon's block, Tenon's capsule is separated from the sclera, and local anaesthetic is instilled into the sub-Tenon's/episcleral space. To be most effective, the anaesthetic must diffuse back to the posterior globe near the optic nerve. Here the posterior ciliary nerves perforate Tenon's capsule and pass through Tenon's space to penetrate sclera (Figure 1). These nerve branches originate from the ophthalmic division of the trigeminal nerve as the long posterior ciliary nerves and, as non-synapsing fibres, pass through the ciliary ganglion, coursing forward as the short posterior

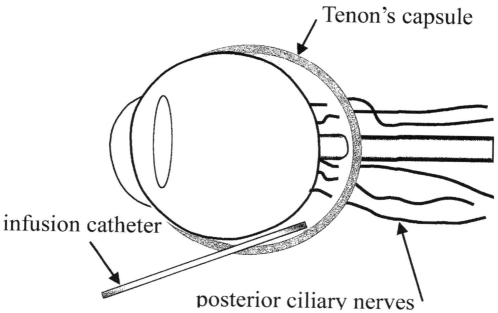

Fig. 1. Sub-Tenon's infusion with catheter placed beneath Tenon's capsule. The anaesthetic agent is injected and diffuses to the posterior ciliary nerves.

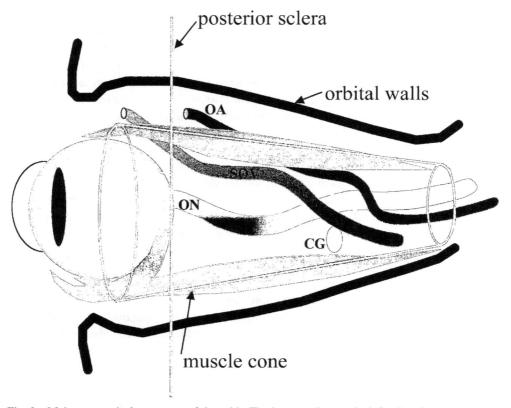

Fig. 2.   Major anatomical structures of the orbit. The intraconal space is defined as the compartment
bounded by the four rectus muscles.

ciliary nerves. They are the sensory nerve supply from the ciliary body, iris, and
cornea. In addition, the short posterior ciliary nerves carry postsynaptic parasympathetic motor fibres from the Edinger-Wesphal nucleus to the ciliary body and
iris. Placement of sufficient local anaesthetic into the posterior Tenon's space will
provide both sensory and motor blockade to the anterior intraocular structures.

The potential complications of the sub-Tenon's block are injury to the globe and
to the vessels and nerves that traverse the episcleral space.

Relevant Orbital Anatomy

One needs to have a visual picture of the major anatomic structures and their relationships during ocular movement. This visual, or 'eidetic' image allows the surgeon
or anaesthetist to navigate the orbit with greater confidence.

From an anatomical perspective the orbit can be visualised as having two major
compartments, the extraconal space and the intraconal space. The intraconal space is
defined as the compartment roughly bounded by the four rectus muscles, from the
annulus of Zinn at the orbital apex, to their penetration through Tenon's capsule (Figure
2). Although there is an extensive system of orbital fascial membranes interconnecting

the muscles and suspending them to the orbital walls, nevertheless, the classic notion of an encircling membrane (the intermuscular septum) separating the two compartments is a conceptual convenience more than an anatomic reality.[26,27] Local anaesthetic and other fluids can easily diffuse from the extraconal space into the intraconal compartment, which explains the efficacy of both intraconal and extraconal placement of anaesthetic agents,[28] and the rapid distribution of haemorrhage throughout the orbit. The addition of hyaluronidase to the local anaesthetic agent may help diffusion across the interlobular septal membranes, enhancing the anaesthetic effect, and reducing the need for supplemental blocks.[29]

Within the orbit, larger vascular and neural elements are concentrated in the orbital apex, and these diverge as they extend forward. Thus, the greatest density of structures at greatest risk for injury is in the apical one-third of the orbit, approximately 32 to 44 mm behind the orbital rim. This is the region where the ciliary ganglion is located and where cranial nerves III, IV and VI penetrate their respective extraocular muscles. The vortex veins, ophthalmic artery, superior and inferior ophthalmic veins, and the muscular arteries are also concentrated here. However, except for the inferior ophthalmic vein, its venous plexus, and the ciliary ganglion and nerves, most of these structures are situated in the superior half of the orbit. Therefore, a 32-mm or less needle inserted into the inferolateral intraconal space offers the lowest risk to these structures. Anatomically, entry into the superior or superomedial orbit carries the highest risk of injury.

In the posterior orbit, situated between the lateral rectus muscle and the optic nerve, is the ciliary ganglion where parasympathetic fibres destined for the ciliary body and iris synapse. This is also the region of the orbit where the motor nerves to the extraocular muscles penetrate the conal surface of the muscles (Figure 3). Local anaesthetic agents placed in this region will produce both sensory and motor blockade and frequently produce amaurosis. A low-volume block will generally not provide sensory block to the eyelids since these branches of the trigeminal nerve primarily run in the superior extraconal space and lie within the bony infraorbital canal in the floor. Thus, if eyelid surgery is contemplated, a greater volume of local anaesthetic must be given or additional regional or local blocks may be required. Of great concern is the central retinal artery located near the ciliary ganglion and entering the optic nerve on its inferior aspect. Injury to this small vessel will result in blindness.

The length of the orbit and the relative location of other anatomic structures is highly variable. Katsev et al.[30] measured the depth of the normal orbit and the position of the ciliary ganglion in cadaver specimens. They showed that the average distance from the inferolateral orbital rim to the apex is 48 mm, with a range of 42 to 54 mm. Similar findings were reported by Karampatakis et al.[31] The annulus of Zinn, enclosing the optic nerve, extends 8 to 9 mm in front of the orbital apex so that this immobile and more vulnerable portion of the nerve can lie as little as 33 mm from the orbital rim in the shortest orbits. Katsev et al. also showed that the average distance from the rim to the ciliary ganglion was 38 mm, with a range of 32 to 44 mm.[30]

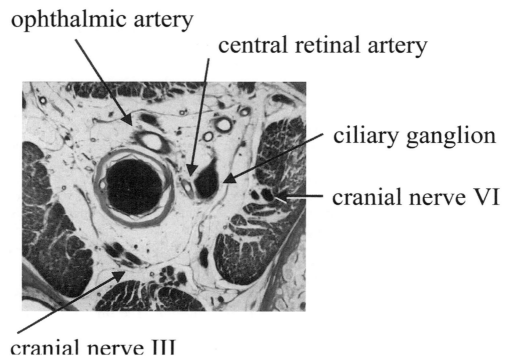

ophthalmic artery

central retinal artery

ciliary ganglion

cranial nerve VI

cranial nerve III

Fig. 3.   Histological section through the posterior inferolateral orbit in the region containing the ciliary ganglion.

Using a 40-mm retrobulbar needle, Karampatakis et al found that in 100% of cadaver specimens studied, the needle tip reached the posterior optic nerve, and in nearly 60% (7/12) it significantly pushed against the nerve.[32] Even when utilizing a 35-mm needle, the tip engaged the optic nerve sheath in 18% of cases. It is clear, therefore, that, in order to ensure a safe approach to the orbital apex and ciliary ganglion, a retrobulbar needle should not exceed 32 mm in length.

Anatomy of Ocular Movement

Of significant interest to the surgeon or anaesthetist delivering orbital anaesthesia is the relative shift in position of the major anatomic structures with movement of the eye. Knowledge of these relationships can allow us to utilise the safe zones for passage of the retrobulbar needle and to shift certain structures into less vulnerable positions.

On looking up, the optic nerve and ciliary ganglion are displaced downward into the inferior orbit, and the inferior oblique muscle is displaced forward towards the orbital rim (Figure 4). This position lessens the risk of injury to the muscle and makes it easier to achieve sensory blockade at the ciliary ganglion. However, it puts the optic nerve closer to the orbital floor and therefore at greater risk of penetration.

Looking down, the optic nerve and ciliary ganglion are displaced upward, and the inferior oblique muscle is shifted backward (Figure 5). This puts the muscle closer

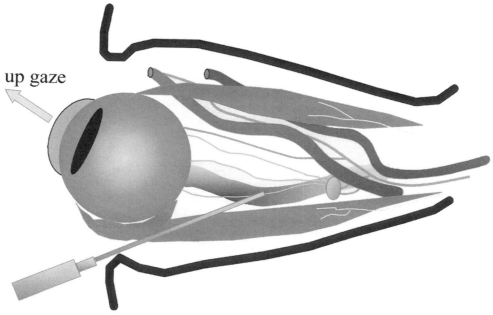

Fig. 4. Shift in the position of orbital structures when the globe is looking up.

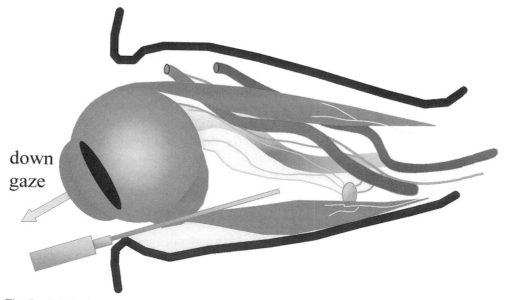

Fig. 5. Shift in the position of orbital structure when the globe is looking down.

to the mid-orbital floor and well behind the orbital rim and therefore into the potential path of the retrobulbar needle. However, this is the safest position to prevent injury to the optic nerve.

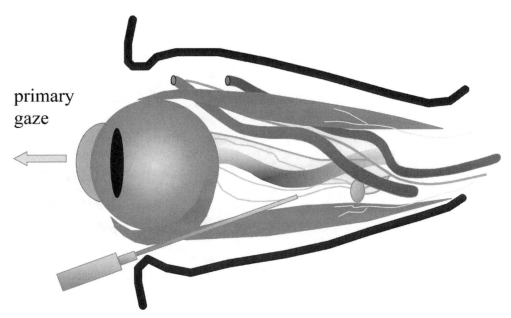

primary
gaze

Fig. 6.   Position of orbital structures and the retrobulbar needle when the globe is in the primary gaze
          position.

The primary gaze position offers a good compromise between optic nerve and inferior oblique muscle positions (Figure 6). It also avoids having the patient look directly at the needle and thus reduces apprehension. In this position the retrobulbar needle can be introduced at the inferolateral orbital rim and advanced parallel to the floor to the level of the posterior globe. It must be kept in mind that the posterior globe position depends on many factors and can be highly variable among patients. The relative degree of proptosis or shallowness of the orbit can significantly alter the depth of the globe within the orbit, as can the degree of myopia and globe size.[33] The posterior sclera can vary from less than 10 mm behind the orbital rim to more than 18 mm. In patients with orbital diseases, such as Graves' disease, or in those with marked enophthalmos from trauma, this disparity can be even greater. A careful evaluation of the globe in relation to the orbital rims will help determine the probable depth of the posterior pole.

When the advancing retrobulbar needle reaches the depth of the posterior surface of the globe, the needle must be directed slightly upward. At this point the bony orbital floor slopes upward to the apex at an angle of about 10 to 15 degrees. In the traditional retrobulbar injection, the needle tip is advanced into the intraconal space between the lateral and inferior rectus muscles to reach the vicinity of the ciliary ganglion. As mentioned above, this region of the orbit is relatively devoid of vascular structures and therefore provides some degree of safety. In the peribulbar block, the anaesthetic is injected within the extraconal space without penetrating the muscle cone. In the mid-orbit the rectus muscles lie about 5 mm from the orbital walls so that this space is quite narrow. Also, along the inferolateral wall lies the inferior orbital fissure containing Müller's orbital muscle and a highly vascular network of penetrating venules passing to the pterygopalatine venous plexus. Injury here can cause significant orbital bleeding.

Conclusion

It should be clear that the placement of a needle and injection of local anaesthetic into the orbit is not a procedure to be taken lightly, or to be casually performed by the novice. Whilst the vast majority of procedures proceed uneventfully, the risks are significant and the potential complications can be devastating. Techniques that minimize these risks are available, both as modifications to the classic retrobulbar block, or as one of the newer, 'less invasive' techniques. However, regardless of the specific technique employed, it behoves the anaesthesia operator to understand the major components of orbital anatomy and their contributions to potential complications.

References

1   Jacobi PC, Dietlein TS, Jacobi FK. A comparative study of topical vs retrobulbar anesthesia in complicated cataract surgery. *Arch Ophthalmol.* 2000; 118:1037–1043.
2   Shomaker ST, Pace NL, van Eerd A, Clinch T. A comparison of topical and retrobulbar anesthesia for cataract surgery. *Ophthalmology.* 1996; 103:1196–1203.
3   Leaming DV. Practice styles and preferences of ASCRS members-1998 survey. *J Cataract Refract Surg.* 1999; 25:851–859.
4   Troll GF. Regional ophthalmic anesthesia: safe techniques and avoidance of complications. *J Clin Anesth.* 1995; 7:163–172.
5   Edge R, Navon S. Scleral perforation during retrobulbar and peribulbar anesthesia: risk factors and outcome in 50,000 consecutive injections. *J Cataract Refract Surg.* 1999; 25:1237–1244.
6   Brooks HL, Brown GC, Federman JL, Fischer DH, Tasman WS. Inadvertent globe perforation during retrobulbar and peribulbar anesthesia: Patient characteristics, surgical management, and visual outcome. *Ophthalmology.* 1991; 98:519–526.
7   Mount AM, Seward HC. Scleral perforations during peribulbar anaesthesia. *Eye.* 1993; 7:766–767.
8   Antworth MV, Hammer ME, Roseman RL. Perforating ocular injuries caused by anesthetic personnel. *Ophthalmology.* 1991; 98:1011–1016.
9   Rivera AH. Needle penetration of the globe during retrobulbar and peribulbar injections. *Ophthalmology.* 1991; 98:1017–1024.
10   Bullock JD, Warwar RE, Green WR. Ocular explosion during cataract surgery: a clinical, histopathological, experimental, and biophysical study. *Trans Am Ophthalmol Soc.* 1998; 96:243–276.
11   Peterson WC, Yanoff M. Complications of local ocular anesthesia. *Int Ophthalmol Clin.* 1992; 32(4):23–30.
12   Davis DB, Mandel MR. Efficacy and complication rate of 16,224 consecutive peribulbar blocks. *J Cataract Refract Surg.* 1994; 20:327–337.
13   Baguneid S, Edge KR. Central nervous system complications after 6000 retrobulbar blocks. *Anesth Analg.* 1987; 66:1298–1302.
14   Javitt JC, Addiego R, Friedberg HL, Libonati MM, Leahy JJ. Brainstem anesthesia after retrobulbar block. *Ophthalmology.* 1987; 94:718–723.

15   Rosen WJ. Brainstem anesthesia presenting as dysarthria. *J Cataract Refract Surg.* 1999; 25:1170–1171.
16   Jackson K, Vote D. Multiple cranial nerve palsies complicating retrobulbar eye block. *Anaesth Intensive Care.* 1998; 26:662–664.
17   Ando K, Ohira A, Takao M. Restrictive strabismus after retrobulbar anesthesia. *Jpn J Ophthalmol.* 1997; 41:23–26.
18   Salama H, Farr AK, Guyton DL. Anesthetic myotoxicity as a cause of restrictive strabismus after scleral buckling surgery. *Retina.* 2000; 20:478–482.
19   Schacher S, Luthi M, Schipper I. Vertical diplopia after cataract operation. *Klin Monatbl Augenheilk.* 2000; 216:295–297.
20   Avilla CW, Braverman DE, Greenhaw ST, Green ME, McCartney DL, Tabin GC. Cluster of diplopia cases after periocular anesthesia without hyaluronidase. *J Cataract Refract Surg.* 1999; 25:1245–1249.
21   Corboy JM, Jiang X. Postanesthetic hypotropia: a unique syndrome in left eyes. *J Cataract Refract Surg.* 1997; 23:1394–1398.
22   Hamilton RC, Gimbel HV, Strunin L. Regional anesthesia for 12,000 cataract extraction and intraocular lens implantation procedures. *Can J Anaesth.* 1988; 35:615–623.
23   Cionni RJ, Osher RH. Retrobulbar hemorrhage. *Ophthalmology.* 1991; 98:1153–1155.
24   Girard LJ. Subperiosteal orbital hemorrhage from retrobulbar injection resulting in blindness. *Arch Ophthalmol.* 1997; 115:1085–1086.
25   Hulbert MF, Yang WC, Pennefather PM, Moore JK. Pulsatile ocular blood flow and intraocular pressure during retrobulbar injection of lignocaine: influence of additives. *J Glaucoma.* 1998; 7:413–416.
26   Dutton JJ. *Clinical and surgical orbital anatomy.* WB Saunders Company, Philadelphia, 1994. 93–111.
27   Koornneef L. The architecture of the musculo-fibrous apparatus in the human orbit. *Acta Morphol Neerl Scand.* 1977; 15:35–64.
28   Prat-Pradal D, Vivien B, Eledjam JJ. Peribulbar versus retrobulbar anesthesia for ophthalmic surgery: An anatomical comparison of extraconal and intraconal injections. *Anesthesiology.* 2001; 94:56–62.
29   Kallio H, Paloheimo M, Maunuksela EL. Hyaluronidase as an adjuvant in bupivacaine-lidocaine mixture for retrobulbar/peribulbar block. *Anesth Analg.* 2000; 91:934–937.
30   Katsev DA, Drews RC, Rose BT. An anatomic study of retrobulbar needle path length. *Ophthalmology.* 1989; 96:1221–1224.
31   Karampatiakis V, Natsis K, Gigis P, Stangos NT. Orbital depth measurements of human skulls in relation to retrobulbar anesthesia. *Eur J Ophthalmol.* 1998; 8:118–120.
32   Karampatakis V, Natsis K, Gigis P, Stangos NT. The risk of optic nerve injury in retrobulbar anesthesia: a comparative study of 35 and 40 mm retrobulbar needles in 12 cadavers. *Eur J Ophthalmol.* 1998; 8:184–187.
33   Modarres M, Parvaresh MM, Hashemi M, Peyman GA: Inadvertent globe perforation during retrobulbar injection in high myopes. *Int Ophthalmol.* 1997; 21:179–185.

3

Ocular Physiology

Mr. B.B. Patil
Mr. T.C. Dowd

Aims and Objectives

This chapter will cover the physiology of the eye that might be relevant to a clinical ophthalmic anaesthetist.

Intraocular Pressure (IOP)

Intraocular pressure is the tension exerted by the contents of the globe on the corneoscleral envelope. The normal intraocular pressure lies in a range between 10 and 20 mm Hg. There is, in general, an increase in IOP with age.[1] IOP is equal between the sexes in ages 20–40 years.[1] There is a positive correlation between IOP and axial length of the globe.[1] There is a diurnal variation of 2–3 mm Hg, with higher pressures in the morning than in the evening. The IOP may differ by as much as 5-mm Hg between the two eyes. IOP increases when changing from the sitting to the supine position, with reported average pressure differences of 0.3–6.0 mm Hg.[1] Transient rises in IOP are seen with coughing, straining or vomiting, and are of no consequence to the intact eye. However, a prolonged rise in IOP is detrimental to the eye causing progressive loss of field of vision.

Aqueous Humour

Composition of Aqueous
Aqueous is a clear fluid that fills the anterior and posterior chambers of the eye. Its volume is about 250 µl and is produced at a rate of 2.5 µl/min. The composition of aqueous is similar to that of plasma except for a much higher concentration of ascorbate, pyruvate and lactate; and a lower concentration of protein, urea and glucose.

Dynamics

IOP is a function of the rate at which aqueous humour enters the eye (inflow) and the rate at which it leaves the eye (outflow). When inflow equals outflow, the pressure remains fairly constant. Inflow is related to the rate of aqueous humour production, whilst outflow depends on the resistance to the flow of aqueous from the eye and the pressure in the episcleral veins. The control of IOP, therefore, is a function of:

a.   production of aqueous humour;
b.   resistance to aqueous humour outflow; and
c.   episcleral venous pressure.

Production

Aqueous is derived from plasma within the capillary network of the ciliary processes by the following mechanisms:

a.   diffusion (transport of lipid-soluble substances through the lipid portions of the membrane proportional to the concentration gradient across the membrane);
b.   ultrafiltration (transport of water and water-soluble substances in response to an osmotic gradient or hydrostatic pressure);
c.   secretion (water soluble substances that are actively transported across the cell membrane).

Outflow

Aqueous produced by the ciliary processes enters the posterior chamber (space between the iris and anterior surface of the lens) and leaves the eye via the trabecular meshwork in the anterior chamber angle into the Schlemm's canal. Schlemm's canal is connected to episcleral and conjunctival veins by a complex system of vessels. The episcleral veins, via the anterior ciliary and superior ophthalmic veins, drain into the cavernous sinus. This outflow pathway, referred to as the 'Conventional System', accounts for 83–96% of aqueous outflow in human eyes.[1] The other 5–15% of aqueous leaves the eye by a number of other systems that are partially understood, namely, uveoscleral and uveovortex systems.[1] Collectively these are called the 'Unconventional System.' Normal episcleral venous pressure is in the range of 8–11 mm Hg.[1] Any sudden increase in episcleral venous pressure, such as that produced by a Valsalva manoeuvre will result in an immediate rise in IOP. Engorgement of the intraocular vessel volume, principally the choroidal vessels and a decreased pressure head for aqueous outflow may explain this rise in IOP.[2]

Factors Affecting IOP

Arterial Blood Pressure

A sudden rise in systemic blood pressure would seem to cause a rise in IOP due to an increase in blood flow through the choroidal vessels. However, studies[3] in cats have shown that an increase in systemic blood pressure does result in pressure changes in the ophthalmic artery, but this is poorly transmitted to the rest of the circulation in the eye. Blood flow in the human eye remains constant over a range of perfusion pressures due to autoregulation of retinal and choroidal circulation. A reduction in systemic arterial blood pressure reduces IOP but this does not become significant until the systemic blood pressure is reduced to <90 mm Hg.[4] A decrease in choroidal blood volume is thought to cause the fall in IOP. Hypotension leads to reduced perfusion of the ciliary body and subsequently decreases aqueous production.[5]

Venous Pressure

Venous congestion caused by coughing, straining, vomiting or Valsalva increases the intraocular vessel volume and decreases the episcleral venous drainage, thus causing a rise in IOP. Head tilt up decreases venous congestion and reduces the IOP and head down tilt causes venous pooling and subsequently a rise in IOP.[6]

Arterial Blood Gases

The partial pressures of carbon dioxide (pCO_2) and oxygen (pO_2) affect the intraocular vascular tone and thus the IOP. A rise in pCO_2 due to hypoventilation results in dilatation of the choroidal vessels and a rise in IOP. Conversely, a fall in pCO_2 causes constriction of the choroidal vessels and a fall in IOP.[7] Hypoxia causes dilatation of intraocular vessels and thus increases IOP; hyperoxia has a constricting effect on the intraocular vessels thus decreasing the IOP. Metabolic acidosis reduces IOP and metabolic alkalosis increases IOP.

Drugs

In general, drugs such as narcotics, hypnotics, major tranquillizers, volatile anaesthetic agents are associated with a fall in IOP, with the exception of ketamine.[8] The effect of depolarising and non-depolarising muscle relaxants on IOP have frequently been investigated, with the common finding that the former causes a small, transient but consistent rise in IOP and the latter consistently produces no change or reduction in IOP if other factors are standardised. Anaesthetic drugs may reduce IOP either by a:

- direct effect on the central diencephalic control centre;
- reduction of aqueous production;
- facilitation of aqueous drainage;
- relaxation of extraocular muscle tone.

Local Anaesthesia

Changes in IOP after peribulbar and retrobulbar injections have been investigated and there is a definite and variable rise in IOP following the start of peribulbar injection.[9] The increase in IOP is transient and depends on the rate and volume of injection.

General Anaesthesia

The effect of drugs has already been discussed. Physical intervention by the anaesthetist may also affect IOP. Laryngoscopy and intubation are associated with a rise in IOP.[10] The insertion of a laryngeal mask airway (LMA) is also associated with a rise in IOP[11] but not to the degree associated with traditional laryngoscopy and intubation. Extubation accompanied by coughing or gagging on the endotracheal tube is associated with a rise in IOP.

Tear Film

The tear film is a protective covering for the cornea. The functions of tear film are:

1. It contributes to the smooth optical properties of the corneal surface.
2. It regulates hydration of the cornea.
3. It is the primary source of oxygen for the cornea.
4. It acts as a lubricant between the lids and the corneal surface.
5. It protects the surface against infection because of the antibacterials lactoferrin, lysozyme, and betalysin.
6. The flushing action of tears across the ocular surface removes exfoliating cells, debris and foreign bodies.
7. It plays a role in healing of central wounds of the avascular cornea, providing a pathway for white blood cells to reach the central cornea from the limbal and conjunctival circulation.

The tear film is composed of three layers:

a. superficial lipid layer;
b. middle aqueous layer;
c. deep mucin layer.

The lipid layer is derived from the meibomian glands (modified sebaceous glands). This layer serves to:

- retard evaporation from the tear film;
- lubricate the action of the lids;
- prevent migration of skin lipids to the ocular surface;
- thicken and stabilize the tear film;
- prevent tear overflow.

The aqueous layer forms the bulk of the tear film and is produced by the main and accessory lacrimal glands. It contains immunoglobulins (IgA, IgG), proteins (e.g., lactoferrin and lysozyme) and electrolytes, which contribute to its antibacterial, antiadhesive and lubricant properties.

The innermost mucin layer is produced by the goblet cells of the conjunctiva and consists of hydrated glycoproteins. It stabilizes the overlying aqueous layer by providing a hydrophilic contact surface.

Tear Outflow

Approximately 25% of secreted tears are lost by evaporation and 75% are pumped into the nasal cavity through the lacrimal drainage system. In most age groups, the lower cannaliculus is responsible for the drainage of approximately 60% of the tear volume. The action of blinking spreads the tears over the cornea, moves them towards the puncti and pumps them through the canaliculi into the lacrimal sac. General anaesthesia reduces the production and stability of tears.[12]

Eyelids

The functions of the eyelids are to:

1.   protect the eye from exposure;
2.   regulate the amount of light entering the eye;
3.   maintain the physical portion of the globe in the orbit;
4.   aid in tear drainage.

Loss of blinking action results in corneal exposure and a subsequent degradation of the health of its surface.[13]

Cornea

The cornea is a clear transparent tissue. The following factors are thought to be responsible for its clarity:

1.   avascularity;
2.   non-keratinised surface epithelium;
3.   the regular arrangement of epithelial and endothelial cells;
4.   a state of relative corneal dehydration which is maintained by an endothelial pump mechanism.

The cornea provides the eye with a clear refractive media, tensile strength and protection from external factors. It is richly supplied by sensory nerves and is probably the most sensitive tissue in the body. Corneal nerves, in addition to serving as sensory receptors, are also responsible for the well being of the surface corneal epithelium. Patients with sensory denervation of the cornea, for example as in diabetes mellitus or herpes simplex infection, suffer from a high incidence of corneal abrasions and ulcers. Failure of the eyelids to close completely (lagophthalmos) during the perioperative period can result in corneal drying and corneal epithelial defects.

Eye Movements

The four recti and the two obliques comprise the extraocular muscles and contribute to eye movements. The levator palpebrae superiorus muscle of the upper lid is also an anatomical member of the extraocular muscles.

Types of eye movements:

- Ductions — monocular movements.
- Versions — binocular, conjugate movements in same direction.
- Vergences — binocular, disconjugate movements in opposite direction.

Conjugate eye movements are classified as:

- Saccades — rapid fast conjugate shifts of gaze from one fixation point to another. The function of saccades is to place the object of interest on the fovea rapidly.
- Smooth pursuit — slow conjugate movements to maintain the object of regard on or near the fovea.

Vergence is further classified as:

- Convergence — ability of the eyes to turn inward.
- Divergence — ability of the eyes to turn outwards from a convergent position.

Control of Eye Movements

Eye muscles are in a state of tonic activity when the eyes are looking straight ahead (primary gaze).

The pathway for saccadic movements originates in the premotor cortex of the frontal motor area (Figure 1). From there, fibres pass to the contralateral horizontal gaze centre in the paramedian pontine reticular formation (PPRF). The right frontal lobe controls saccades to the left and the left frontal lobe those to the right. Irritating lesions may therefore cause a deviation of the eyes to the opposite side away from the irritation. From the horizontal gaze centre (PPRF) the output is to the ipsilateral abducens nucleus to abduct the ipsilateral eye. To adduct the contralateral eye some fibres from PPRF cross the midline and pass through the medial longitudinal fasciculus (MLF) to reach the contralateral medial rectus nucleus via the third nerve complex. Stimulation of the PPRF on one side therefore causes a conjugate movement of eyes to the same side. The PPRF also receives inputs from cerebellum, basal ganglia, vestibular nuclei and cervical proprioceptors giving rise to fine and accurate gaze control. The control of vertical saccades is not as clearly anatomically defined as its horizontal counterpart. The vertical gaze centre is located in the rostral interstitial nucleus of the MLF in the midbrain. From each vertical gaze centre, impulses pass to the subnuclei of the eye muscles controlling vertical gaze in both eyes. The vertical centre has no identifiable cortical control.

Pursuit movements are generated in the ipsilateral occipito-parietal area, so that the right hemisphere controls a pursuit movement to the right. Little is known of the neuronal pathway.

The final common motor pathway occurs via the III, IV and VI cranial nerves supplying the extraocular muscles.

Saccadic eye movements can be used to test for the residual effects of anaesthesia.[14] Varying depths of anaesthesia cause variations in muscle tone. This can affect

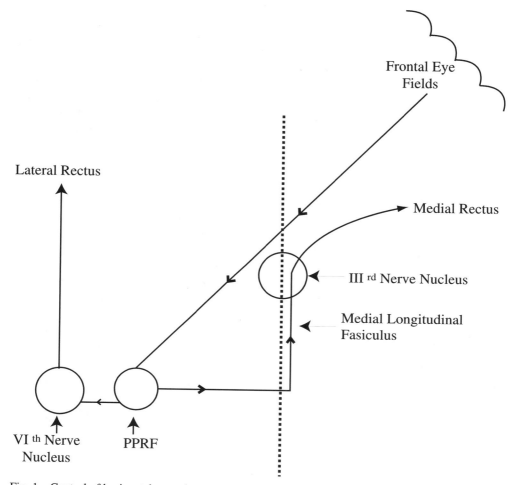

Fig. 1. Control of horizontal saccades.

the results of the forced duction test done by surgeons during strabismus surgery. In this test, the corneoscleral junction is held by forceps and the eye is moved in all fields of gaze so as to differentiate a paretic muscle from mechanical restriction. For this reason, some surgeons prefer neuromuscular blockade whilst performing the test.[15]

Under physiological conditions, vestibular stimulation occurs from head movements. The resulting slow eye movements, known as vestibular ocular responses (VOR), compensate for the head motion such that the position of the eyes in space remains static and steady visual fixation can be maintained. The 'doll's head manoeuvre' is a clinical method of testing the VOR. The patient is asked to fixate on a target whilst the examiner moves the head in a horizontal or vertical plane. A normal response consists of a conjugate eye deviation in the direction away from head rotation such that the eyes remain stable with respect to space despite the head movement. In unconscious patients this test may be used as a method of assessing eye movements and thus brainstem function. The pathway is a three-neuron connection from the vestibular neuron through the vestibular nucleus directly to the contralateral horizontal gaze centre. Another way to stimulate the vestibular system is by caloric irrigation. Cold water irrigation into the auditory canal induces a predominantly horizontal jerk nystagmus with a fast phase opposite to the side of irrigation, and warm water irrigation induces a similar jerk nystagmus with a fast phase toward the side of irrigation. (The mnemonic device is 'COWS': Cold opposite, Warm same).

Oculocardiac Reflex (Aschner's Reflex)

Aschner[16] and Dagnini[17] first described the oculocardiac reflex in 1908. Sinus bradycardia, nodal rhythm, ectopic beats or sinus arrest occurs due to pressure, torsion or traction on the extraocular muscles. It is a trigemino-vagal reflex; the afferent arc is via the long and short ciliary nerves to the ciliary ganglion, the ophthalmic division of trigeminal nerve, terminating in the main sensory nucleus of the trigeminal nerve in the floor of the fourth ventricle. The efferent impulses pass down the vagus nerve. This reflex occurs both in adults and children, but is seen more commonly in children. This may be because of the higher frequency of squint surgery in this age group.
   Retrobulbar anaesthesia may block the conduction at the ciliary ganglion (afferent limb) and intravenous atropine sulphate blocks the peripheral muscarinic receptors at the heart (efferent limb).[18] Premedication with atropine, prior to general anaesthetic, reduces the incidence and the morbidity of the oculocardiac reflex.[19] Grover et al[20] showed that local anaesthesia produced less bradycardia and ectopic arrhythmia and therefore may be safer than general anaesthesia for adult surgery in which traction of the extraocular muscles is required.

Oculo-respiratory Reflex

Petzetakis[21] reported the oculo-respiratory reflex in humans. This reflex consists of shallow breathing, slowing of the respiratory rate or full respiratory arrest. The afferent pathways are similar to the oculocardiac reflex. It is postulated that a connection exists between the trigeminal sensory nucleus and the pneumotaxic centre in the pons and the medullary respiratory centre. This reflex is commonly seen in strabismus surgery. Atropine has no effect on this reflex. In a spontaneously breathing patient this reflex may lead to hypoxemia and hypercarbia if not recognised promptly. It is therefore suggested that controlled ventilation should be employed for all children undergoing squint surgery.[22]

The Oculo-emetic Reflex

This reflex is thought to be responsible for the high incidence of vomiting (60–90%) after squint surgery. It is a trigemino-vagal reflex, the stimulus being the pulling of the extraocular muscle. Antiemetics may slightly reduce its incidence.

Periocular anaesthesia, which blocks the afferent arc, may seem to be the best approach in prevention.

Pupil

The size of the normal pupil varies at different ages, from person to person, and with different emotional states, level of alertness, degrees of accommodation and ambient room light. The normal pupillary diameter is 3–4 mm, is smaller in infancy, and tending to be larger in childhood and again progressively smaller with advancing age. The excursion of the pupil can be extraordinarily large, from 1 mm to 9 mm.[23] Approximately 20% of the normal population have unequal pupils[23] (anisocoria). This pupillary inequality is not constant in an individual; it may decrease or increase, or reverse sides within days or hours. A healthy iris is moving all the time even when illumination and accommodation are constant. This physiological unrest is called 'hippus.' It is presumed to be due to fluctuations in the activity of the sympathetic and parasympathetic innervation of the iris muscles.

The iris contains two muscles, the sphincter and the dilator muscle. They are innervated by the autonomic nervous system. The parasympathetic nerve fibres derived from the oculomotor nerve supply the sphincter muscle. These are postganglionic fibres that travel to the eye from the ciliary ganglion via the short ciliary nerves). Non-myelinated sympathetic fibres innervate the dilator muscle. The pre-ganglionic neuron cell bodies are situated in the lateral grey horn of the first thoracic segments of the spinal cord and its fibres relay in the superior cervical ganglion. Postganglionic fibres leave the superior cervical ganglion along the carotid plexus, traverse the nasociliary branch of ophthalmic division of the trigeminal nerve and via the long ciliary nerve to reach the dilator muscle. Thus parasympathetic stimulation causes constriction and sympathetic stimulation causes dilatation of the pupil.

Functions of Pupil

- Regulates the amount of light entering the eye.
- Increases the depth of focus for near vision.
- Reduces optical aberration.

Light Reflex

The pathway for the pupillary light reflex commences in the retinal ganglion cells, enters the optic nerve, decussates at the optic chiasm and traverses the optic tract (Figure 2). It leaves the tract before the lateral geniculate body (LGB) and synapses in the pretectal nucleus in the mid-brain. Fibres from the pretectal nucleus go to both the Edinger-Westphal nuclei (thus there are two decussations — once in the chiasm and once again in the Edinger-Westphal nuclei). Parasympathetic fibres from the Edinger-Westphal nucleus travel along cranial nerve III synapse in the ciliary

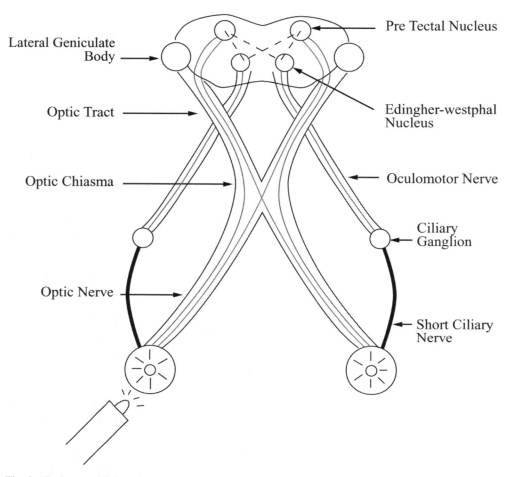

Pre Tectal Nucleus

Lateral Geniculate
Body

Optic Tract

Edingher-westphal
Nucleus

Optic Chiasma

Oculomotor Nerve

Ciliary
Ganglion

Optic Nerve

Short Ciliary
Nerve

Fig. 2.   Pathway of light reflex.

ganglion, then, via the short ciliary nerves, supply the sphincter muscle. Light shown in one eye thus gives rise to bilateral and symmetrical pupillary constriction.

Pupillary responses to light can be direct and indirect (consensual). The direct light reflex occurs when the pupil constricts to the light shown directly into the eye and indirect occurs when light shown in one eye produces constriction of the pupil in the other eye.

Afferent Pupillary Defects
The pupil of an eye that is blind from retinal or optic nerve disease fails to react to light shown directly, but constricts consensually when the light is shown in the other (healthy) eye. The blind eye is then said to have an 'afferent pupillary defect'. This happens because the pupillomotor stimulus from the blind eye is diminished when compared to the healthy eye.

Efferent Pupillary Defects
Poor reaction to light occurs when the parasympathetic supply to the iris sphincter is impaired. The pupil would appear to be dilated and fixed if the damage is anywhere along its efferent pathway.

Accommodation-convergence Reaction (Near Reflex)
The near reflex is a synkinetic reflex consisting of pupillary constriction (miosis), convergence and accommodation.

Visual Acuity

Visual acuity is defined as the power of the eye to resolve two stimuli separated in space. A variety of tests are necessary to test acuities in different age groups. There are tests for infants, children and adults, both for literates and illiterates. The most common test used is the Snellen chart. The smallest line of letters read by the patient, when viewed at 6 metres is noted. The test distance over the smallest line of letters seen gives the visual acuity. It is a common misconception that periocular anaesthesia blocks all the optic nerve conduction and that the patient doesn't see anything. In fact, some optic nerve function can be retained and the patients' vision can be anywhere between no perception of light to seeing the operating microscope. Proper preoperative counselling of patients in this respect can help reduce patient anxiety.

Colour Vision

Colour vision is a function of the cones (a type of photoreceptor cell in the retina). There are three main types of cones, one each for the three primary colours; red, green and blue. Any colour can be matched by using these three primaries. The density of the cones falls sharply outside the fovea. The centre of the fovea has the highest density of cones, mainly red and green, whilst the blue cones are outer to these. Cones are also responsible for vision in lit conditions (photopic vision), whilst rods (another type of photoreceptor cell in the retina) are responsible for vision in the dark (scotopic vision).

A minimum requirement for colour discrimination is the presence of at least two kinds of cone photopigment and normal colour vision requires the presence of all three.

Colour Blindness

Colour blindness can be defined as a diminished ability to perceive differences in colour. It can be congenital or acquired. Congenital colour blindness affects males more than females (8% versus 0.5%) and is inherited as X-linked recessive gene. It almost always is of the 'red–green' variety and both eyes are equally affected. On the other hand, the acquired type of colour blindness has an equal incidence in both sexes, usually is of the 'blue–yellow' variety and more commonly affects one eye more than the other.

Anomalous Trichromatism

This is the most common type of colour blindness. These individuals require three primaries for matching an unknown colour but — unlike normal trichromats — use them in anomalous amounts. Thus protans use more red; deutans more green; and tritans more blue.

Dichromatism

These are individuals whose photoreceptors contain only two of the three cone photopigments. Protanopes lack red; deuteronopes green; and tritanopes blue.

Monochromatism

This is of two types; both forms leave the affected individual completely without colour discrimination.

a.   Rod monochromatism: The individual is born without functioning cones in the retina. This occurs in 1:30,000 of the population. Individuals with this condition have low visual acuity, absent colour vision, photophobia and nystagmus.

b.   Cone monochromatism: Affected individuals do have cones but all the cones contain the same visual pigment. This is a rare condition, occurring in 1:100,000. These individuals have normal visual acuity but cannot discriminate coloured lights of equal luminosity.

Tests for Colour Vision

Normal colour vision requires healthy functioning of the macula and optic nerve. The most common testing technique utilises a series of polychromatic plates, such as those of Ishihara or Hardy-Rand-Rittler. The plates are made up of dots of the primary colours printed on a background mosaic of similar dots in a confusing variety of secondary colours. The primary dots are arranged in simple patterns (numbers or geometric shapes) that cannot be recognized by patients with deficient colour perception.

References

1   Shields, MB. In: *Textbook of glaucoma*, 4th ed. Williams & Wilkins, Baltimore, 1998. pp 14, 25, 47–49.

2   Hart WM. Intra-ocular pressure. In: Hart WM Jr, editor. *Alders's physiology of the eye*. 9th ed. Mosby Year Book, St Louis, 1992. p 257.

3   Macri FJ. Vascular pressure relationships and the intra-ocular pressure. *Arch Ophthalmol*. 1961; 65:571–574.

4   Adams AK, Barnett KC. Anaesthesia and IOP. *Anaesthesia*. 1961; 21:202–210.

5   Forrest FC. Ocular physiology relevant to anaesthesia. In: Johnson RW, Forrest FC, editors. *Local and general anaesthesia for ophthalmic surgery*. Butterworth- Heinemann, Oxford, 1994:4.

6   Tsamparlakis J, Casey TA, Howell W, Edridge A. Dependence of IOP on induced hypotension and posture during surgical anaesthesia. *Trans Ophthalmol Soc UK*. 1980; 100:521–526.

7   Samuel JR, Beaugie A. Effect of CO_2 on the IOP in man during general anaesthetic. *Br J Ophthalmol.* 1974; 58:62–67.

8   Cunningham AS, Barry P. Intra-ocular Pressure – Physiology and implications for anaesthetic management. *Can Anaesth Soc J.* 1986; 33:195–208.

9   Soloman R, Liu C, Sarkies N. IOP changes after peribulbar injection with or without compression. *Br J Ophthalmol.* 1996; 80:394–397.

10   Wynands JF, Cromwell DF. Intra-ocular tension in association with succinylcholide and endotracheal intubation. A preliminary report. *Can Anaesth Soc J.* 1960; 7:39–43.

11   Lamb K, James MF, Janicki PK. The laryngeal mask airway for intra-ocular surgery: effects on IOP and stress response. *Br J Anaesth.* 1992; 69:143–147.

12   White E, Crosse MN. The aetiology and prevention of perioperative corneal abrasions. *Anaesthesia.* 1998; 53:157–161.

13   Hart WM. Eyelids. In: Hart WM Jr, editor. *Alders's physiology of the eye.* 9th ed. Mosby Year Book, St Louis, 1992. p 1.

14   Paut O, Vercher, JL, Blin O, Lacarelle B, Mestre D, Durand A, Grautier GM, Lambu-lines J. Evaluation of saccadic eye movements as an objective test of recovering from anaesthesia. *Acta Anaesthsiol Scan.* 1995; 39(8):1117–1124.

15   Dell R, Williams B. Anaesthesia for strabismus surgery, a regional survey. *Br J Anaesth.* 1999; 82:761–763.

16   Aschner B. Uber bisher noch nicht beschribenen Reflex von Auge auf Krieslauf und Atmung: Verschinden des Radialispulses bei Druk auf das Auge. *Wien Klin Wochenschr.* 1908; 1529–1530.

17   Dagnini G. Intorno ad un riflesso provocato in alcuni emiplegici collo stimolo della cornea e colla pressione sul bulbo oculare. *Boll Sci Med.* 1908; 8:380–381.

18   Misurga VK, Singh SP, Kulshrestha VK. Prevention of oculocardiac reflex during extra-ocular muscle surgery. *Indian J Ophthalmol.* 1990; 38:85–87.

19   Chong JL, Tan SH. Oculocadiac reflex in strabismus surgery under general anaesthetic – A study of Singapore patients. *Singapore Med J.* 1990; 31:38–41.

20   Grover VK, Bhardwaj N, Shabana N, Grewal SP. Oculocardiac reflex during retinal surgery using peribulbar block and nitrous narcotic anaesthesia. *Ophthalmic Surg Lasers.* 1998; 29:207–212.

21   Petzetakis M. Effects reflexes de la compression oculaire a l'etat normal. Reflexes oculo-cardiaque, oculo-respiratoire, oculo-vasomoteur. *J Physiol (Paris).* 1915; 16:1027–1048.

22   Blanc F, Jacob J, Milot J, Cryenne L. The oculorespiratory reflex revisited. *Can J Anaesth.* 1998; 35:468–472.

23   H. Stanley Thompson. The pupil. In: Hart WM Jr, editor. *Alders's physiology of the eye.* 9th ed. Mosby Year Book, St Louis, 1992. pp 412–414.

4

Pharmacology for Regional Ophthalmic Anaesthesia

Dr Hamish A. McLure

Introduction

In ophthalmic surgery the anaesthetist and surgeon have ample opportunity to cause sight-threatening injuries. By the injection of highly concentrated, potentially toxic solutions into frail elderly patients, the anaesthetist is also well placed to initiate life-threatening systemic injury. Unlike most other regional anaesthetic techniques the injected solution is often a cocktail of several agents. The 'backbone' ingredient is one of several local anaesthetics, or a mixture of local anaesthetics, with adjuvants to improve speed of onset, spread and duration. This diversity generates extra interest for the enthusiast but may bewilder the occasional practitioner. In addition, the process of mixing agents affords even accomplished anaesthetists another opportunity to inadvertently concoct a toxic solution. In the same way that a better understanding of orbital anatomy may reduce mechanical complications, a greater knowledge of the pharmacology of local anaesthetic solutions may reduce pharmacological iatrogenic complications.

Physiochemical Properties of Local Anaesthetics

Molecular Structure

The molecular structure of local anaesthetics conforms to a similar configuration of lipophilic and hydrophilic portions, connected by a hydrocarbon chain (Figure 1). The lipophilic portion is generally an unsaturated aromatic ring derived from benzoic acid or less commonly from aniline. The hydrophilic moiety is a tertiary or quaternary amine. The bond that links the hydrocarbon chain to the lipophilic moiety may be used to classify the local anaesthetic as an ester, amide, ketone or ether. This classification is not entirely inclusive. Other molecules may have local anaesthetic properties,

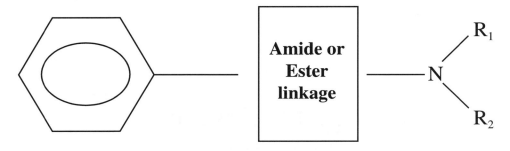

Lipophillic aromatic ring   Hydrophillic amine

Fig. 1. Structure of local anaesthetics.

although they are seldom used for ophthalmic regional anaesthesia. In practice it is the amide and ester compounds that may be found in the hospital formulary. The ester bond is relatively unstable compared to the others, readily undergoing hydrolytic cleavage. The reduced stability ensures rapid metabolism in vivo. In vitro, shelf life is dramatically reduced and autoclave sterilisation of ampoules is impossible.

Ionisation

Local anaesthetics are weak bases (pK_a 7.6–8.9), poorly soluble in water and therefore usually constituted in acidic hydrochloride salt solutions (pH ~ 6). In an acidic environment the local anaesthetic accepts a hydrogen ion and becomes charged. This process is rapidly reversible and a dynamic equilibrium is established with the proportion of ionised to un-ionised varying with the solution pH and pK_a of that agent (Figure 2). The relationship between the pH, agent pK_a and quantities of ionised to un-ionised is represented by the Henderson–Hasselbach equation:

$$pK_a = pH + Log\ (BH^+ / B)$$

$$B\quad +\quad H^+\ \rightleftharpoons\ BH^+$$

Fig. 2. Dynamic equilibrium between ionised and un-ionised local anaesthetic.

The pK_a represents the pH at which ionised and un-ionised drug are present in equal masses. The clinical relevance of the pK_a is in its relationship to speed of onset. The un-ionised form is able to penetrate the highly lipid cell membrane, but once inside the cell it is the ionised form which is active. Most of the commonly used local anaesthetics have pK_a values around 8 (Table 1). Consequently, at normal physiological pH of 7.4, local anaesthetics exist predominantly in the ionised form that is unable to penetrate the cell. Those with lower pK_a values will have a comparatively greater proportion in the neutral form and thus will diffuse more rapidly across the membrane and have a faster onset of action. Increasing the pH of the carrier solution increases the proportion of un-ionised local anaesthetic, reducing the time of onset. The penalty is less chemical stability with the risk of precipitation.

Table 1. Physiochemical and clinical properties of local anaesthetics.

Agent	pK_a (25° C)	Speed of onset	Partition coefficient[1]	Potency	Toxicity	Protein bound (%)	Duration
Amide agents							
Bupivacaine	8.1	intermediate	346	high	high	95	long
Levobupivacaine	8.1	intermediate	346	high	intermediate	96	long
Etidocaine	7.7	fast	800	high	high	94	long
Lidocaine	7.7	fast	43	intermediate	low	64	intermediate
Mepivacaine	7.6	fast	21	intermediate	low	75	intermediate
Prilocaine	7.8	fast	25	intermediate	low	55	intermediate
Ropivacaine	8.2	intermediate	115	intermediate	intermediate	94	long
Ester agents							
Cocaine	8.7	slow	U[2]	high	very high	98	long
Amethocaine	8.5	slow	221	intermediate	intermediate	76	intermediate
Procaine	8.9	slow	1.7	low	low	6	short

[1] Partition coefficients with n-octanol/buffer, [2] U Unknown

Inflammation reduces the tissue pH. The acidic environment drives the equilibrium towards the ionised state reducing the amount available to penetrate the nerve. The clinical result is a weaker block. For this reason and the risk of spreading infection, ophthalmic blocks are contraindicated in the presence of local infection.

Lipid Solubility

The lipid solubility of a local anaesthetic depends upon the aromatic group and length of the hydrocarbon chain. It is quantified by measurement of the relative distribution of the local anaesthetic between an aqueous phase (e.g. buffer at physiological pH) and a non-ionised solvent phase (e.g. octanol, hexane, heptane etc). The partition coefficient (P) corresponds to the relative concentrations of ionised or unionised forms between the two phases, whereas the distribution coefficient (Q) describes the total amount of drug in each phase. As the values of P and Q increase so does the concentration of that local anaesthetic within the nerve membrane, increasing its local anaesthetic action. Consequently, lipid solubility is the major determinant of local anaesthetic potency. Bupivacaine and etidocaine have the greatest lipid solubility and potency, followed by lidocaine and mepivacaine, with procaine the least lipid soluble and least potent agent.

Protein Binding

Local anaesthetics bind to tissue and plasma proteins (albumin, α_1-acid glycoprotein). It is the unbound 'free' local anaesthetic that is active, whilst the protein-bound drug acts as a reservoir, prolonging the duration of action. As local anaesthetics are administered, the protein binding sites become occupied with little change in unbound plasma concentration. Once the proteins are saturated there may be a sudden, precipitous rise in free local anaesthetic with rapid onset of the symptoms and signs of toxicity. This may also occur if plasma pH falls, causing dissociation of local anaesthetic from protein molecules with an increase in free fraction and potential toxicity. Clinically, if a patient's general condition deteriorates after a dose of local anaesthetic they may develop local anaesthetic toxicity much later than expected, delaying the additional diagnosis.

Chirality

Molecules with asymmetric carbon atoms may exist in mirror image isomeric forms. They are differentiated and labelled according to the direction they deflect polarised light as S-(-)-laevorotatory or R-(+)-dextrorotatory. Bupivacaine, etidocaine, mepivacaine, prilocaine and ropivacaine all have asymmetric carbons. Most are produced as racemic mixtures (equal numbers of S- and R-isomers), with the exception of ropivacaine, which is synthesised as the chirally pure S-isomer. The S-isomer of bupivacaine (levobupivacaine) has also been marketed separately from the racemic mixture. These isomers have identical lipid solubility and ionisation characteristics, but may behave very differently at biological receptors. S-bupivacaine and S-ropivacaine have similar local anaesthetic properties but markedly reduced toxicity compared to their R-isomeric forms. The exception is etidocaine where the isomers behave identically.

Physiology of Nerve Conduction

Impulses are propagated along the nerve by transient changes in permeability of the membrane to sodium. In the resting state the membrane is impermeable to sodium. A sodium–potassium pump actively moves sodium out of the cell in exchange for potassium. The intracellular potassium concentration is high compared to extracellular fluid. As the membrane is relatively permeable to potassium, some leaks out along a concentration gradient. The active movement of sodium coupled with leakage of potassium generates a polarised membrane with a trans-membrane electrical potential difference of −70 to −90 mV.

Stimulation of the nerve causes conformational changes in membrane lipoprotein sodium channels, which switch from a closed to an open state. This results in a sudden influx of sodium ions along an electrochemical gradient, raising the membrane potential. If sufficient channels open and the membrane potential reaches a threshold value (−60 mV) then widespread opening of sodium channels occurs, and the membrane potential rises (depolarisation) to around +20 mV. There is a brief period during which the sodium channel is inactive and relatively refractory. The leakage of potassium and active pumping of sodium then restores the membrane potential to its polarised state.

Once an area of axon has been depolarised the intracellular portion has a positive charge relative to adjacent areas of nerve, producing a flow of ions and generating an electrical current. The change in potential within the adjacent areas causes sodium channels to open and further depolarisation occurs. A wave of depolarisation then flows along the nerve propagating the original stimulus. The inactive refractory period prevents rapid re-depolarisation of the area originally affected and inhibits retrograde conduction of the impulse.

Mechanism of Action of Local Anaesthetics

Local anaesthetics reversibly block sodium channels by interfering with their ability to undergo conformational changes. Gradually increasing the concentration of local anaesthetic reduces the rate of rise of the action potential, eventually preventing impulse transmission. It is the ionised form of the local anaesthetic that binds to and obstructs the intracellular portion of the sodium channel. The unionised form may also act within the membrane, causing a disorganised expansion and disruption of the membrane and sodium channel. Local anaesthetics have differing affinities for the sodium channel depending on the state of the channel. Affinity is maximal when the sodium channel is either open or inactive but reduced when the channel is closed. Binding to the channel is cyclical with attachment during the open and inactive phases, followed by dissociation when the channel is closed. There are significant differences in the rate of dissociation. Lidocaine dissociates quickly whereas R-bupivacaine dissociates slowly, with ropivacaine intermediate. In nerve cells this is unimportant as the cyclical changes in the sodium channel are rapid. However, in cardiac fibres the cyclical changes are considerably slower. Lidocaine dissociates rapidly preventing a frequency-dependent blockade, but R-bupivacaine dissociates sufficiently slowly to allow a frequency-dependent blockade to develop leading to arrhythmias and myocardial depression. In general the slower the rate of dissociation the more likely that local anaesthetic is to produce toxic myocardial side effects.

Metabolism and Excretion of Local Anaesthetics

Ester local anaesthetics are hydrolysed very rapidly by cholinesterase in the tissues and plasma. The speed of degradation lends a degree of safety as plasma levels fall quickly. Patients with cholinesterase deficiency may be at increased risk of toxicity due to reduced rate of hydrolysis. The metabolites of hydrolysis are inactive. However, metabolism of procaine yields p-amino benzoic acid, an antigen causing allergic reactions. The exception to plasma hydrolysis is cocaine, which undergoes metabolism in the liver.

Amide local anaesthetics are systemically absorbed then distributed, initially to the pulmonary circulation. The low pH of lung extravascular tissue compared to plasma causes ion trapping in the lung. This temporary sequestration blunts the sudden increase in plasma levels that would otherwise occur after a bolus dose. Distribution and uptake of local anaesthetic by the other tissues are dependent upon the binding affinity of the agent to plasma proteins and other blood-borne sites (e.g. on erythrocytes), tissue binding affinity and lipid solubility. Amide local anaesthetics are stable in blood and are cleared mainly by liver metabolism, with a small fraction by renal excretion. Liver microsomal enzymes transform the local anaesthetic into less active and inactive metabolites. The rate of metabolism differs between agents with prilocaine and etidocaine being the most rapid, lidocaine and mepivacaine intermediate, with ropivacaine then bupivacaine the slowest. There is no correlation between rate of metabolism and lipid solubility, potency or protein binding. The clearance of prilocaine exceeds that possible with liver blood flow indicating that there are other sites of metabolism, most probably the lung. Again there are differences between the stereoisomers of the local anaesthetics. R-bupivacaine, the more toxic form, is cleared 20% faster from the plasma than the S-isomer. In contrast, there appears to be no difference between the isomers of prilocaine.

Toxicity

This may be local direct toxicity to nerves within the orbit or the intraorbital muscles, or it may be systemic toxicity from excessive absorption or intravascular or dural injection.

Local Toxicity

Neurotoxicity
If injected directly into nerves, or in situations where highly concentrated local anaesthetic bathes nerves for prolonged periods, local anaesthetics may be neurotoxic. Laboratory studies have demonstrated this even in the lower concentrations used in clinical practice.[1] Clinically, the use of spinal microcatheters and 5% lidocaine has been associated with cases of prolonged neuronal damage.[2] In ophthalmic regional anaesthesia neither the concentration of the local anaesthetic nor the duration of exposure are excessive, so the local anaesthetic alone is unlikely to be a cause of neurological dysfunction. However, highly concentrated local anaesthetic in association with vasoconstrictors, high orbital pressures and coexistent vascular pathology may give rise to nerve ischaemia and damage.

Myotoxicity
Direct injection of local anaesthetics into muscle can induce muscle necrosis. Subsequent healing with fibrosis and contracture may impair muscle function sufficiently to require surgery. The muscles most often involved are the inferior oblique and inferior rectus (inferotemporal injection) and the medial rectus (medial canthus injection). Prolonged muscle palsy is devastating for elderly patients. The practitioner must understand orbital anatomy and avoid direct intramuscular injections.

Systemic Toxicity
Systemic complications are seldom seen, but they present significant risks. They may follow toxic reactions caused by elevated plasma levels of local anaesthetic or follow subarachnoid injections where plasma levels are normal. The latter occur when the dural cuff ensheathing the proximal optic nerve is pierced and a sufficient dose of local anaesthetic is administered into cerebrospinal fluid in continuity with that bathing the cerebral hemispheres and brainstem. This presents with loss of consciousness, respiratory depression and hypotension. Treatment is aimed at maintaining oxygenation with positive pressure ventilation and the use of fluids and

vasopressors until the local anaesthetic effect has subsided. Toxic reactions affect the central nervous systems (CNS) and cardiovascular system. They occur most frequently after inadvertent intravascular injection but rarely may follow overdose, rapid systemic absorption or intraarterial injection with retrograde flow to the brain and brainstem.

CNS Reactions

These occur at lower plasma levels than cardiovascular reactions. They may present with tongue and perioral tingling, progressing to dizziness, restlessness, confusion, muscle twitching, convulsions, coma and respiratory and cardiovascular depression.

Cardiovascular Reactions

Cardiovascular toxicity usually follows CNS toxicity, although there are reports of precipitous cardiac reactions occurring without any prodromal CNS symptoms.[3] The cardiovascular effects tend to be biphasic, starting with tachycardia, hypertension and a variety of arrhythmias, progressing to cardiovascular depression. Virtually any arrhythmia can occur from multi-focal ectopics, through to ventricular tachycardia, ventricular fibrillation and asystole.

Treatment of CNS and cardiovascular toxic reactions is supportive. Oxygenation must be maintained with the use of supported ventilation, anticonvulsants, fluids, vasopressors and antiarrhythmics where necessary. Systemic toxicity associated with bupivacaine or etidocaine is often refractory to treatment.[3] Resuscitation is likely to be prolonged, so it is essential that careful attention is paid to developing hypoxia, acidosis or electrolyte derangement as these will make a successful outcome less likely. Concerns about bupivacaine toxicity have driven the development and marketing of S-bupivacaine and S-ropivacaine. Animal and human volunteer studies have demonstrated their reduced CNS and cardiac toxicity compared to their R-isomeric forms.[4–8]

Adjuvants

In an attempt to modify the speed of onset, duration and quality of block adjuvants may be added to the local anaesthetic solution. The evidence for their effectiveness is often conflicting, a reflection of the multifactorial nature of the quality of block. With this in mind it is important to 'do no harm' when introducing an adjuvant that may have only marginal effects on the quality of the intended block. Mistakes may easily be made in the preparation of these cocktails and so great caution must be exercised.

Hyaluronidase

Hyaluronidase, an ovine testicular protein, hydrolyses extracellular hyaluronic acid, thereby degrading the ground substance that bonds cells together. It is added in varying concentrations to the local anaesthetic solution to promote greater spread, improving the block and minimising the increase in orbital pressure. As noted in other regional techniques, the evidence for the efficacy of hyaluronidase is conflicting. Some investigators have found it to be useful in concentrations as low as 7.5 iu ml^{-1}, whereas others have been unable to demonstrate any beneficial effect with concentrations as high as 150 iu ml^{-1}.[9–12] This apparent discord may be the result of failure to standardise the pH of the injectate. Hyaluronidase works best over the relatively narrow pH range of 6.4–7.4. However, different local anaesthetic solutions with varying additives may have very different pH values. Attempts to tease out the usefulness of hyaluronidase with any given local anaesthetic solution are frequently hampered by the failure of study groups to standardise, or even record, the pH of the test solutions. Despite these difficulties there are some striking results. Roberts found that addition of hyaluronidase 10 iu/ml alone to a lidocaine/bupivacaine/adrenaline mixture (pH 3.9) made no difference to the block nor did alkalinisation (pH 5.1).[13] However, addition of hyaluronidase and alkalinisation (pH 6.7) significantly improved the quality of block. Side effects are rare, although hyaluronidase has been implicated in allergic reactions and the formation of an orbital pseudotumour.[14]

Vasoconstrictors
Local anaesthetics tend to exert a vasodilator action, depending on the local anaesthetic, the concentration and stereoisomer, vascular responsiveness and blockade of autonomic pathways. However, for the highly concentrated local anaesthetics used in ophthalmic anaesthesia the predominant effect is vasodilatory. Vasoconstrictors reduce orbital perfusion, minimising washout of local anaesthetic and prolonging the duration of action. In addition, the quality of block may be improved, orbital volume and therefore pressure reduced and peak (potentially toxic) plasma levels are decreased.[15]

Epinephrine is the most commonly added vasoconstrictor. The commercially prepared solutions contain sodium metabisulphite (an allergen) and are highly acidic to improve the stability of epinephrine. Similarly to hyaluronidase, pH manipulation may be required to fully exploit the potential of epinephrine with these solutions. Many anaesthetists prefer to add epinephrine immediately before injection. The resulting solution has a higher pH and thus should be less painful and better able to penetrate the tissues. The desired concentration is 5 μg ml^{-1} (1 in 200,000), which can be made up by adding 0.1 ml of 1 in 1000 epinephrine to 20 ml of local anaesthetic. Great care should be exercised as higher concentrations may have a systemic effect or critically impair globe perfusion. Even with the standard concentration solutions there have been concerns about the reduction in retinal perfusion. Colour Doppler ultrasound has been used in a primate model to demonstrate significant decreases in retinal perfusion pressure when retrobulbar injections with 2% lidocaine with epinephrine (5 μg ml^{-1}) solutions were performed.[16] This has been confirmed in human subjects undergoing retrobulbar anaesthesia, which in itself reduces retinal perfusion by increasing orbital pressure.[17] The link between the use of vasoconstrictors and subsequent retinal pathology has not been demonstrated. However, it would seem wise to avoid these additives in patients with known vascular problems.

pH Manipulation

Raising the pH of local anaesthetic solutions by adding sodium bicarbonate will increase the proportion of non-ionised base. This should result in improved onset time and duration of regional anaesthetic block, which has been demonstrated for sciatic, brachial plexus and epidural blocks. The evidence for use in ophthalmic regional anaesthesia is conflicting, with some authors achieving marked improvements and others seeing little or no benefit.[18,19]

Whilst pH manipulation aims to alter the amount of un-ionised base available to penetrate the nerve, the process of carbonation aims to increase the amount of ionised base generated within the nerve. Carbon dioxide is added to the local anaesthetic solution. It is intended to diffuse into the cell, generate carbonic acid, lowering the pH thereby increasing the proportion of ionised local anaesthetic close to its site of action. Although theoretically promising, and successful in the laboratory, carbonation has not proved reliable clinically and so is not in widespread use.

Other Additives

Reah[20] added 0.5 mg vecuronium to a 10-ml mixture of 0.75% bupivacaine, 2% lidocaine and 15 iu ml^{-1} hyaluronidase with 5 μg ml^{-1} epinephrine. In comparison to a control group who received no vecuronium, the study group showed significantly better globe and lid akinesia. However, this technique has not gained popular acceptance.

Low dose morphine has been added to mixtures of local anaesthetics for retrobulbar blockade in the hope of stimulating peripheral opiate receptors.[21] As has been observed when opiates were used for other regional anaesthetic techniques, the results have suggested that the opiates are more likely to be acting centrally.

Clonidine, an alpha-2-adrenoreceptor agonist, has also been added to local anaesthetic mixtures with varying degrees of success. Mjahed[22] added 2 μg/kg of clonidine to 3–4 ml of 2% lidocaine for retrobulbar blockade and found that it caused a decrease in intraocular pressure and increased the duration of analgesia and akinesia. These results were not replicated by Connolly,[23] who added 100 μg clonidine to 7 ml 1% lidocaine for peribulbar blockade and found no significant differences with respect to pain, akinesia or intraocular pressure.

Choice of Local Anaesthetic

The aims of ophthalmic regional anaesthesia are to provide high-quality analgesia, akinesia and globe hypotonia. The process should be quick, painless and last for the duration of surgery without being excessively prolonged. To reduce orbital pressure the ideal agent should have vasoconstrictor properties, be able to penetrate tissues easily and be potent enough to require minimal volumes. In addition, it should have a wide margin of safety in terms of systemic, neuro- and myotoxicity. The perfect agent has yet to be found. However, in high concentration virtually any of the currently available local anaesthetics can provide adequate conditions for ophthalmic surgery. The topical application of local anaesthetic alone is a popular technique in some centres, but usually a combination of topical followed by orbital injections is used.

Topical Local Anaesthetics

Cocaine
Despite its virtual disappearance from the ophthalmic theatre, no discussion about local anaesthetics, particularly for ophthalmic regional anaesthesia, would be complete without mention of cocaine. Cocaine, an ester of benzoic acid, found naturally in the leaves of *Erythroxylon cola*, has been used recreationally and medicinally for hundreds of years. It rose to prominence in 1884 when Carl Koller, an ophthalmic surgeon in Vienna, noted the local anaesthetic action of cocaine when instilled into his own conjunctiva. This event marked the discovery of local anaesthesia and was the birthplace of modern regional anaesthetic practice. Initial enthusiasm for the use of deep orbital injections of cocaine to enable more invasive surgery soon disappeared as reports of systemic toxicity and death were published. Cocaine not only acts as a local anaesthetic but also inhibits the reuptake of norepinephrine at sympathetic neurones, which potentiates the effects of catecholamines. Excessive systemic absorption of cocaine leads to hypertension, tachycardia, tachypnoea, nausea and a myriad of central nervous systems side effects. Despite this unappealing toxicity profile, cocaine is a popular drug of abuse. It took the relatively recent introduction of safer local anaesthetics before ophthalmic regional anaesthesia began to flourish. In the UK the use of cocaine tends to be limited to that of being a topical agent with vasoconstrictor properties for procedures involving the nasal mucosa.

Amethocaine (Tetracaine)
Amethocaine, an ester and analogue of procaine, is highly potent. The 1% solution is popular in the UK for topical anaesthesia. Like most of the other topical agents its onset of action is quick (around 20 seconds), and the duration of action is up to 20 minutes. Its main disadvantages are that it stings and is relatively toxic to the cornea.

Oxybuprocaine (Benoxinate)
Oxybuprocaine 0.4% is an ester local anaesthetic used exclusively for topical anaesthesia. It is a popular choice as it is less painful with decreased corneal toxicity compared to amethocaine.

Proxymetacaine (proparacaine)
Proxymetacaine is a less irritant local topical anaesthetic usually presented in a 0.5% solution. It has a shorter duration of action than the others. It is not particularly antigenic and is useful in patients who are sensitive to the amide local anaesthetics.

Local Anaesthetics used for Orbital Injections

Bupivacaine (Marcain)

Bupivacaine, the butyl derivative of a ringed piperidine carboxylic acid amide, was introduced in 1963. Despite concerns about toxicity, bupivacaine has remained a popular choice for regional anaesthesia due to its high potency and long duration of action. Adequate sensory blockade may be achieved with 0.5% bupivacaine, but 0.75% solution is more reliable to achieve adequate akinesia. With the higher concentration solution the onset of block is similar to that with 2% lidocaine, but the duration is significantly prolonged. Although superficially attractive this may lead to diplopia the day following surgery, which is a disabling handicap for elderly patients. In one study 70% of patients who had received 0.75% bupivacaine had a persistent block and diplopia the day following surgery, compared to just 8% who had received a mixture of 0.75% bupivacaine and 2% lidocaine.[24] Lidocaine is often added to hasten the onset and reduce the potential toxicity of the large dose of local anaesthetic. Surprisingly, lidocaine may confer an additional advantage of raising the threshold for cardiotoxicity caused by the bupivacaine.[25]

Levobupivacaine (Chirocaine)

Levobupivacaine (S-bupivacaine) possesses the same physiochemical properties as R-bupivacaine. In vivo, it has similar anaesthetic potency, but an increased margin of safety with respect to cardiovascular and central nervous system toxic effects.[6,26] A significantly greater amount of levobupivacaine is required to produce cardiac arrhythmias and cardiac arrest compared to racemic bupivacaine, and if one of these crises occurs then resuscitation is more likely to be successful. Levobupivacaine 0.75% has been compared with the racemic mixture for peribulbar anaesthesia and found to be clinically indistinguishable.[27] The improved safety profile is a significant advantage in the vulnerable elderly population who can least tolerate adverse events.

2-Chloroprocaine (Nesacaine)

2-Chloroprocaine, an ester, has a rapid onset, brief duration and low systemic toxicity. It is metabolised four times faster than procaine, its analogue, so is much less toxic. In a small study Cass compared 2% with 3% 2-chloroprocaine for peribulbar anaesthesia and found both provided adequate conditions for cataract surgery, although the duration of action was marginally longer with the higher concentration.[28]

Etidocaine (Duranest)

An amide agent introduced in 1972, etidocaine is used in the US and Scandinavia but is not available in the UK. It is a potent agent with a long duration of action and may be used in concentrations of 0.5–1.5% for ophthalmic regional anaesthesia where it produces a fast onset of dense, prolonged akinesia, but reduced analgesia compared to bupivacaine.[29] Etidocaine suffered adverse publicity alongside bupivacaine when Albright's editorial[3] highlighted the risks of cardiotoxicity in a series of cases, one of whom received a caudal injection of etidocaine.

Lidocaine (Lignocaine, Xylocaine)
Introduced in 1947, lidocaine is a tertiary amide derivative of diethylamino-acetic acid. It is moderately potent with a rapid onset of action. Protein binding is significantly less than with bupivacaine and predictably the duration of action is much shorter. It is commonly used in concentrations up to 2% for orbital injections where it provides anaesthesia for around an hour depending on concentration, volume and additives. It is also used as an infusion for intracameral anaesthesia, often supplemented by topical local anaesthetic drops. Lidocaine has remained a popular choice because it has one of the safest toxicity profiles and is a familiar agent for most clinicians.

Mepivacaine (Carbocaine)
Mepivacaine, introduced in 1957, is unavailable in the UK but is used in the rest of Europe and the US. It is the methyl derivative of a ringed piperidine and is structurally related to bupivacaine, although clinically similar in terms of potency and duration of action to lidocaine. In ophthalmic regional anaesthesia it may be injected in concentrations of 2–3%. Some investigators have found that the addition of epinephrine dramatically prolongs the action of mepivacaine.

Prilocaine (Citanest)
Prilocaine is a secondary amine analogue of lidocaine with similar potency, rapid onset and duration of action. It may be used in concentrations of 2–4% and, as it is a potent vasodilator, is usually combined with a vasoconstrictor (felypressin). The 3% solution has been compared favourably with 2% lidocaine with epinephrine and 0.5–0.75% bupivacaine mixed with 2% lidocaine for peribulbar anaesthesia.[30–32] Rapid uptake by tissues and swift metabolism in the liver and lungs lend prilocaine an admirable safety record. A well-known, but rarely seen, side effect is the development of cyanosis with high plasma levels of an aminophenol metabolite. This compound is able to oxidise haemoglobin to methaemoglobin. If the patient becomes symptomatic, high-concentration oxygen and intravenous methylene blue (1 mg kg^{-1}) should be administered. This agent is not licensed for ophthalmic use in the UK.

Prilocaine may also be mixed with lidocaine in an oil/water emulsion known as EMLA (Eutectic Mixture of Local Anaesthetics). This compound has a very low melting point such that it is a cream at room temperature. It is able to penetrate skin remarkably easily and thus has been used in ophthalmic regional anaesthesia as an adjunct technique to reduce the pain of needle insertion for deep orbital injections.[33]

Ropivacaine (Naropin)
Ropivacaine is structurally related to bupivacaine and mepivacaine and is produced commercially as a solution of the pure S-isomer. Its pharmacodynamic profile is similar to bupivacaine, although with slightly reduced potency. In low concentrations there appears to be a differential sensory-motor block with a degree of motor sparing. However, a dense motor block is desirable in ophthalmic surgery, so for peribulbar anaesthesia 0.75–1% ropivacaine is used. The resulting blocks are comparable to those found with 0.75% bupivacaine with 2% lidocaine, although the mixture has

slightly more rapid an onset of akinesia.[34–36] The advantage of ropivacaine is reduced cardiovascular and CNS toxicity. However, as bupivacaine and ropivacaine are not equipotent some of this advantage may be lost as larger doses of ropivacaine are required.

References

1   Kanai Y, Katsuki H, Takasaki M. Lidocaine disrupts axonal membrane of rat sciatic nerve in vitro. *Anesth Analg.* 2000; 91:944–948.

2   Schell R, Brauer F, Cole D, Applegate, R. Persistent sacral nerve root deficits after continuous spinal anaesthesia. *Can J Anaesth.* 1991; 38:908–911.

3   Albright G. Cardiac arrest following regional anesthesia with etidocaine or bupivacaine. *Anesthesiology.* 1979; 51:285–287.

4   Vanhoutte F, Vereecke J, Verbeke N, Carmeliet E. Stereoselective effects of enantiomers of bupivacaine on the electrophysiological properties of guinea pig papillary muscle. *Br J Pharmac.* 1991; 103:1275–1281.

5   Valenzuela C, Snyders D, Bennet P, Tamargo J, Hondeghem L. Stereoselective block of cardiac sodium channels by bupivacaine in guinea pig ventricular myocytes. *Circulation.* 1995; 92:3014–3024.

6   Huang Y, Pryor M, Mather L. Cardiovascular and central nervous system effects of intravenous levobupivacaine and bupivacaine in sheep. *Anesth Analg.* 1998; 86:797–804.

7   Pitkanen M, Feldman H, Arthur G, Covino B. Chronotropic and inotropic effects of ropivacaine, bupivacaine and lidocaine in the spontaneously beating and electrically paced isolated, perfused rabbit heart. *Reg Anesth.* 1992; 17:183–192.

8   Knudsen K, Beckman M, Blomberg S, Sjovall J, Edvardsson N. Central nervous and cardiovascular effects of i.v. infusions of ropivacaine, bupivacaine and placebo in volunteers. *Br J Anaesth.* 1997; 78:507–514.

9   Nicoll J, Treuren B, Acharya P, Ahlen K, James M. Retrobulbar anesthesia: the role of hyaluronidase. *Anesth Analg.* 1986; 65:1324–1328.

10 House P, Hollands R, Schuler M. Choice of anaesthetic agent for peribulbar anaesthesia. *J Cataract Refract Surg.* 1991; 17:80–83.

11 Morsman C, Holden R. The effects of adrenaline, hyaluronidase and age on peribulbar anaesthesia. *Eye.* 1992; 6:290–292.

12 Bowman R, Newman D, Richardson E, Callear A, Flanagan D. Is hyaluronidase helpful for peribulbar anaesthesia? *Eye.* 1997; 11:385–388.

13 Roberts J, MacLeod B, Hollands R. Improved peribulbar anaesthesia with alkalinization and hyaluronidase. *Can J Anaesth.* 1993; 40:835–838.

14 Kempeneers A, Dralands L, Ceuppens J. Hyaluronidase induced orbital pseudotumour as a complication of retrobulbar anesthesia. *Bull Soc Belge Ophthalmol.* 1992; 243:159–66.

15 Barr J, Kirkpatrick N, Dick A, Leonard L, Hawksworth G, Noble DW. Effects of adrenaline and hyaluronidase on plasma concentrations of lidocaine and bupivacaine after peribulbar anaesthesia. *Br J Anaesth.* 1995; 75:692–697.

16 Netland PA S S, Harris A. Color Doppler ultrasound measurements after topical and retrobulbar epinephrine in primate eyes. *Invest Ophthalmol Vis Sci.* 1997; 38:2655–2661.

17 Hessemer V, Heinrich A, Jacobi K. Ocular circulatory changes caused by retrobulbar anesthesia with and without added adrenaline. *Klin Monatsbl Augenheilkd.* 1990; 197:470–479.

18 Lewis P, Hamilton RC, Brant R, Loken R, Maltby J, Strunin L. Comparison of plain with pH-adjusted bupivacaine with hyaluronidase for peribulbar block. *Can J Anaesth.* 1992; 39:555–8.

19   Zahl K, Jordan A, McGroarty J, Gotta A. pH-adjusted bupivacaine and hyaluronidase for peribulbar block. *Anesthesiology*. 1990; 72:230–232.
20   Reah G, Bodenham A, Braithwaite P, Esmond J, Menage M. Peribulbar anaesthesia using a mixture of local anaesthetic and vecuronium. *Anaesthesia*.1998; 53:551–4.
21   Hemmerling T, Budde W, Koppert W, Jonas J. Retrobulbar versus systemic application of morphine during titratable regional anesthesia via retrobulbar catheter in intraocular surgery. *Anesth Analg*. 2000; 91:585–588.
22   Mjahed K, el Harrar N, Hamdani M, Amraoui M, Benaguida M. Lidocaine-clonidine retrobulbar block for cataract surgery in the elderly. *Reg Anesth*. 1996; 21:569–575.
23   Connelly N, Camerlenghi G, Bilodeau M, Hall S, Reuben S, Papale J. Use of clonidine as a component of the peribulbar block in patients undergoing cataract surgery. *Reg Anesth Pain Med*. 1999; 24:426–429.
24   Sarvela P, Paloheimo M, Nikki P. Comparison of pH-adjusted bupivacaine 0.75% and a mixture of bupivacaine 0.75% and lidocaine 2%, both with hyaluronidase, in day-case cataract surgery under regional anesthesia. *Anesth Analg*. 1994; 79:35–39.
25   Fujita Y, Endoh S, Yasukawa T, Sari A. Lidocaine increases the ventricular fibrillation threshold during bupivacaine-induced cadiotoxicity in pigs. *Br J Anaesth*. 1998; 80:218–222.
26   Gristwood R, Bardsley H, Baker H, Dickens J. Reduced cardiotoxicity of levobupivacaine compared with racemic bupivacaine (marcaine): new clinical evidence. *Expert Opin Investig Drugs*. 1994; 3:1209–1212.
27   McLure H, Rubin A. A comparison of 0.75% levobupivacaine with 0.75% racemic bupivacaine for peribulbar anaesthesia. *Anaesthesia*. 1998; 53:1160–1164.
28   Cass G, Reynolds W, Lorenzen T, Leach D, Matson D, et al. Randomized double-blind study of the clinical duration and efficacy of Nesacaine-MPF 2% and 3% in peribulbar anesthesia. *J Cataract Refract Surg*. 1999; 25:1656–1661.
29   Sarvela P. Comparison of regional ophthalmic anaesthesia produced by pH-adjusted 0.75% and 0.5% bupivacaine and 1% and 1.5% etidocaine, all with hyaluronidase. *Anesth Analg*. 1993; 77:131–134.
30   Dopfmer U, Maloney D, Gaynor P, Ratcliffe R, Dopfmer S. Prilocaine 3% is superior to a mixture of bupivacaine and lidocaine for peribulbar anaesthesia. *Br J Anaesth*. 1996; 76:77–80.
31   Henderson T, Franks W. Peribulbar anaesthesia for cataract surgery: prilocaine versus lidocaine and bupivacaine. *Eye*. 1996; 10:497–500.
32   Bedi A, Carabine U. Peribulbar anaesthesia: a double-blind comparison of three local anaesthetic solutions. *Anaesthesia*. 1999; 54:67–71.
33   Joyce PW, Sunderraj P, Villada J, Kirby J, Watson A. A comparison of amethocaine cream with lidocaine-prilocaine cream (EMLA) for reducing pain during retrobulbar injection. *Eye*. 1994; 8:465–466.
34   Corke P, Baker J, Cammack R. Comparison of 1% ropivacaine and a mixture of 2% lidocaine and 0.5% bupivacaine for peribulbar anaesthesia in cataract surgery. *Anaesth Intensive Care*. 1999; 27:249–252.
35   Nicholson G, Sutton B, Hall G. Comparison of 1% ropivacaine with 0.75% bupivacaine and 2% lidocaine for peribulbar anaesthesia. *Br J Anaesth*. 2000; 84:89–91.
36   McLure H, Rubin A, Westcott M, Henderson H. A comparison of 1% ropivacaine with a mixture of 0.75% bupivacaine and 2% lidocaine for peribulbar anaesthesia. *Anaesthesia*. 1999; 54:1178–1182.

5

Preoperative Assessment and Evaluation

Dr Marc A. Feldman

Goals of Preoperative Assessment

Good perioperative medical care begins with a thorough preoperative evaluation, the goals of which are to:

1. establish a doctor–patient relationship
2. psychologically prepare the patient
3. obtain informed consent
4. assess risk and
5. plan perioperative management.

Ophthalmic procedures are the most common surgeries performed in the elderly. In 1999, the Medicare program in the USA processed nearly 2 million claims for anaesthetics for cataract surgery.[1] These operations do not require an inpatient stay and do not involve the blood loss and postoperative pain associated with general surgical procedures. Yet, they are not minor procedures. For the patient, ophthalmic surgery can be a major life event. Establishing a professional relationship before surgery can alleviate anxiety and help the patient prepare for surgery. Giving information to the patient is as important as getting information from the patient. The patient needs to know what to expect. An informed patient will be more calm, comfortable, and cooperative.

The patient must give informed consent. The anaesthetist should discuss the planned anaesthetic procedure, the risks, and any alternatives. This need not take more than a few minutes. It should be unhurried. The discussion of risk should be directed to the individual patient with knowledge of their medical history and physiologic status.

A thorough preoperative evaluation may benefit the patient in many ways. General medical screening may find previously unknown conditions, leading to earlier treatment. Known conditions may be discovered to require additional treatment in order to optimise the patient for surgery.[2] The preoperative assessment represents an opportunity not only to modify operative risk but also to address long-term health issues.[3-5] Occasionally patients will be found to be sufficiently ill to require acute medical care.

Preoperative evaluation presents potential problems as well. Rapport within the medical-care team can be strained as differences of opinion regarding patient management arise. There can be inconsistencies in care and approach that can lead to inefficiencies and to confusion and frustration for both the patient and the medical care team. Last minute cancellation for preoperative issues leads to disruption of the operating room schedule.

The preoperative assessment is focused on improving perioperative outcome. Two important factors influencing outcome are the degree of illness of the patient and the degree of stress of the surgical procedure. Patients with severe medical problems present higher risk and require more intensive investigations before surgery. Patients having extensive surgical procedures also require more intensive studies. Preoperative evaluation of the adult ophthalmic patient is undervalued because it involves the preparation for low risk surgery, even though this is in a high-risk patient.

Those undergoing cataract surgery are in their mid-seventies on average, and most have significant risk factors such as diabetes, hypertension, and atherosclerosis. Cataract has been shown to be a marker for increased mortality in the recent Nurses Health Study.

Ophthalmic surgery itself, however, is low-risk. Mortality after ophthalmic procedures is much lower than for the general surgical population.[6-9] Backer et al.[10] found that ophthalmic surgery did not pose the risk of myocardial re-infarction seen with general surgical procedures.[11] Patient illness has less effect on outcome with these procedures. In a study of unanticipated hospital admissions after outpatient ophthalmic surgery, age and ASA class were not significant factors.[12]

Because they are high-risk patients undergoing low-risk surgery, there is controversy regarding the best preoperative management. Some say that because cataract extraction is a low-stress, bloodless procedure, like getting a haircut, no preop evaluation would affect outcome, so none is indicated. A recent large, multicentre trial[13] showed no effect of preoperative blood tests and electrocardiogram on postoperative outcome. Others say that there is minor surgery, but there is no minor anaesthesia. Every patient must receive a full evaluation to include every possible test, to detect any finding, to institute every therapy, and to delay as long as necessary, so that the patient can be in the best medical condition and have the lowest risk.

Appropriate preoperative medical consultation is important. A study of malpractice litigation in cataract surgery found that medical consultation accounted for 16% of the liability. This compared to 17% attributed to either local or general anaesthesia.[14]

It is as unwise to ignore all risk, as it is to attempt to reduce every risk to the lowest conceivable minimum. The goal is to ensure that the patient is an acceptable risk for the proposed anaesthetic and surgery. The medical care team with the informed consent of the patient determines acceptable risk. Unacceptable risks are present if a patient's condition would indicate that admission for medical treatment is required or if a reversible condition would likely lead to a perioperative complication if left untreated.

The goal is to develop guidelines that would encourage consistency of care and minimise disruption to patients and the operating room. The following guidelines are presented after review of the recent literature and published guidelines.

Patient History

The patient history is the first step in preoperative information gathering. Previous hospitalisations and surgical procedures are reviewed with particular attention to allergies and drug sensitivities. Latex allergy is becoming more common and should be specifically addressed. A current medication list is obtained. Patient factors that could influence anaesthetic management include dementia, deafness, language difficulty, restless leg syndrome, obstructive sleep apnoea, tremors, dizziness, and claustrophobia. A preoperative patient questionnaire can be very helpful.[15] A thorough review of the patient history helps perioperative planning and establishes a doctor–patient relationship.

Physical Examination

Physical examination should address the major systems to check for signs of major cardiac or pulmonary decompensation. Particular attention should be paid to positioning issues. Severe scoliosis or orthopnoea can make proper positioning difficult.

Laboratory investigations

No routine screening tests have been shown to be helpful or to improve outcome. Laboratory studies, if needed, should be determined on the basis of the results of the history and physical exam.[16] As a general rule, the tests that a patient needs prior to ophthalmic procedures are the same as that which the patient would require in the absence of a surgical procedure. Tests are chosen where the results are likely to change management. Urgent medical management is obtained for results reaching critical limits.[17]

Electrocardiogram: Indications for requesting an ECG include:

- new chest pain;
- decreased exercise tolerance;
- palpitations;
- near-syncope;
- fatigue;
- dyspnoea;
- tachycardia, bradycardia or an irregular pulse on examination.

Critical results from the ECG that indicate urgent medical management include:

- signs of acute ischaemia or injury;
- malignant arrhythmia;
- complete heart block;
- atrial fibrillation which is new or with a ventricular response greater than 100 beats per minute.

Serum biochemistry: Indications for requesting a serum electrolyte profile include:

- history of severe vomiting or diarrhoea;
- poor oral intake;
- changes in diuretic management;
- arrhythmia;
- signs or symptoms of renal decompensation;
- polydipsia, polyuria, weight loss.

Critical results from the electrolytes that indicate urgent medical management include:

- sodium less than 120 mmol l^{-1} or greater than 158 mmol l^{-1};
- potassium less than 2.8 mmol l^{-1} or greater than 6.2 mmol l^{-1};
- urea nitrogen greater than 104 mg dl^{-1};
- a blood glucose less than 46 mg dl^{-1} or greater than 484 mg dl^{-1}.

Haematocrit/Haemoglobin: Indications for requesting these include:

- a history of bleeding;
- poor oral intake;
- fatigue;
- decreased exercise tolerance;
- tachycardia.

Critical results again that indicate urgent medical intervention include:

- a haematocrit of less than 18% or greater than 61%;
- a haemoglobin less than 6.6 mg dl^{-1} or greater than 19.9 mg dl^{-1}.

Ophthalmic Evaluation

Elements of the ophthalmic evaluation are important for the anaesthesia assessment. The visual acuity of both eyes should be noted. Patients with poor vision in the non-operative eye face much greater potential functional loss with any complication. The patient should be expected to have a higher anxiety level. If the patient is to be patched overnight, the physician should anticipate the increased need for postoperative assistance and care for a temporarily blind patient.

The axial length of the globe should be assessed. When ultrasound measurements are available, the axial length should be noted. If no ultrasound is available, the myopic patient should be assumed to have an increased axial length. If a posterior staphyloma is present, the risks of injection anaesthesia may be dramatically increased.[18] Preoperative glaucoma history, increased intraocular pressure, and increased axial length are important risk factors for suprachoroidal haemorrhage.[19] The risk may be reduced with tighter control of intraoperative heart rate and blood pressure.[20] Preoperative softening with a compression device may also decrease risk.

Cardiovascular Evaluation

Ophthalmic procedures are rarely stressful from a physiological point of view. They do not predispose to cardiovascular complications unlike major vascular procedures. However, many ophthalmic patients are high-risk. Undergoing an ophthalmic procedure certainly would predispose the very ill patient to a cardiovascular event. In general, ophthalmic patients needs to have the kind of cardiovascular evaluation that would be needed even if they were not having an ophthalmic procedure.

The American Heart Association and American College of Cardiology published guidelines for perioperative cardiovascular evaluation for non-cardiac surgery.[21] Ophthalmic procedures such as cataract extraction are specifically identified as low-risk procedures. For these procedures, evaluation is focused on patients with major clinical predictors of risk. These major predictors generally demand intensive management that often results in delay or cancellation of surgery until the cardiac problem is clarified and appropriately treated.

- Recent myocardial infarction with evidence of significant ischaemic risk. The American College of Cardiology defines recent myocardial infarction as less than or equal to 30 days. This is a much shorter period than the 3–6 months that have often been used as a guideline. Indications for coronary angioplasty or coronary revascularisation procedures are the same as if the patient were not having an ophthalmic procedure.
- Unstable or severe angina. This includes Canadian Class III or IV.[22] Class III is defined as marked limitations of ordinary physical activity. Angina occurs on walking one to two blocks on the level or climbing one flight of stairs. Class IV is defined as the inability to carry on any physical activity without discomfort — angina symptoms may be present at rest.
- Decompensated congestive heart failure. These patients normally cannot lie flat for a procedure.
- Significant arrhythmia. These include high-grade atrioventricular block such as complete heart block, symptomatic ventricular arrhythmia, and supraventricular arrhythmias with uncontrolled ventricular rate. A careful evaluation for drug toxicity or metabolic derangement should be done. Indications for cardiac pacing and antiarrhythmic therapy are the same as in the non-operative setting.
- Severe valvular disease. Symptomatic stenotic lesions are associated with severe congestive heart failure and shock. These may require percutaneous

valvotomy or valve replacement. Symptomatic regurgitant lesions can usually be stabilized with medical therapy. Because ophthalmic procedures are not associated with significant bacteraemia, antibiotic prophylaxis is not recommended.[23]

Hypertension

Hypertension is a common problem in ophthalmic patients. Severe hypertension may lead to perioperative complications. Degrees of hypertension have been defined.[24] Stage 3 of severe hypertension is defined as a systolic of 180 mm Hg or more, or a diastolic of 110 mm Hg or more. It would be prudent to reschedule elective procedures in patients with sustained stage 3 hypertension until after at least two weeks of antihypertensive therapy.

Pulmonary Evaluation

Ophthalmic procedures generally require that the patient lie flat comfortably and quietly. If the patient cannot lie flat, or if there is intractable cough, a perioperative complication is more likely. Preoperative risk reduction strategies include cessation of cigarette smoking, treatment of airflow obstruction with bronchodilators or steroids, and administration of antibiotics for respiratory infections.[25]

Patients should be assessed for sleep apnoea. Intravenous sedation is contraindicated in these patients. For some patients, treatment with a mild stimulant such as caffeine can be helpful in keeping them awake and cooperative during a procedure.

Endocrine Evaluation

Diabetes mellitus is very common in the ophthalmic surgical population. It is best if these patients can be done early in the morning with as little disturbance as possible to their usual daily routine. Severe hyperglycaemia and hypoglycaemia are to be avoided.[26] A fasting blood glucose should be checked preoperatively. Insulin therapy should be used, if needed, to keep the blood glucose in the range of 150–250 mg dl^{-1}. The potential for autonomic neuropathy needs to be considered,[27] especially when elevating the patient from the supine position.

Patients on long-term steroid therapy generally do not require 'stress-dose' steroid treatment for ophthalmic surgery.[28] The patient should be given their normal dose of steroid on the day of surgery. The physician should be alert to the occasional patient who may require additional glucocorticoid perioperatively. Unexpected hypotension, fatigue, and nausea may be signs of a patient who needs additional steroid.

Anticoagulation Therapy

Many patients for ophthalmic surgery present taking anticoagulant medications. Perioperative management of anticoagulant medications involves weighing the relative risks of thrombotic vs. hemorrhagic complications.[29] Either of these results can be devastating to the patient.

The risk of thrombotic complications depends on:

1.   The indication for anticoagulation. Serious complications from arterial thromboembolic disease, such as atrial fibrillation or valvular heart disease, are much more common that complications from venous disease, such as deep venous thrombosis.
2.   The risk factors for thromboembolism in the individual, especially if and when the patient had a previous episode of thromboembolism.

The risk of hemorrhagic complications depends on:

1.   The degree of anticoagulation
2.   The hemorrhagic potential of the surgical procedure. Serious hemorrhagic complications are most probable in orbital and oculoplastic surgery, intermediate in vitreoretinal, glaucoma, and corneal transplant and least likely in cataract surgery.

A consensus is developing that cataract surgery may be safely performed whilst maintaining patients on warfarin.[30] For intermediate-risk procedures, stopping warfarin for four days preoperatively is indicated. For high-risk cases for haemorrhage or thrombosis, conversion of warfarin to heparinisation, may be indicated.

Conclusions

Adequate preoperative evaluation is a medical, ethical, and legal duty of the medical care team. Ophthalmic patients are difficult because they are high-risk patients having low-risk surgery. An appropriate preoperative assessment would include the medical testing and management that a patient would need even in the absence of a surgical procedure. The assessment should also include those factors that would change perioperative anaesthetic or surgical plans. Guidelines improve rapport, encourage consistency, and improve smooth functioning of the operating theatre. Outcome studies are needed and will be seen arising over the next several years to guide practice.

References

1   Bierstein K. How much is Medicare spending on anesthesia services? *ASA Newsl.* 2001; 65:28–31.
2   Donlon JV Jr. Local anesthesia for ophthalmic surgery: patient preparation and management. *Ann Ophthalmol.* 1980; 12:1183–1191.
3   King MS. Preoperative evaluation. *Am Fam Physician.* 2000; 62:387–396.
4   Palda V. PRE-OPportunity knocks: a different way to think about the preoperative evaluation. *Am Fam Physician.* 2000; 62:308–311.
5   Hu FB, Hankinson SE, Stampfer MJ, Manson JE, Colditz GA, Speizer FE, Hennekens CH, Willett WC. Prospective study of cataract extraction and risk of coronary heart disease in women. *Am J Epidemiol.* 2001; 153(9):875–881.

6   Petruscak J, Smith RB, Breslin P. Mortality related to ophthalmological surgery. *Arch Ophthalmol.* 1973; 89:106–109.

7   Quigley HA. Mortality associated with ophthalmic surgery. A 20-year experience at the Wilmer Institute. *Am J Ophthalmol.* 1974; 77:517–524.

8   Hovi-Viander M. Death associated with anaesthesia in Finland. *Br J Anaesth.* 1980; 52:483–489.

9   Vacanti CJ, VanHouten RJ, Hill RC. A statistical analysis of the relationship of physical status to postoperative mortality in 68,388 cases. *Anesth Analg.* 1970; 49:564–566.

10   Backer CL, Tinker JH, Robertson DM, Vlietstra RE. Myocardial reinfarction following local anesthesia for ophthalmic surgery. *Anesth Analg.* 1980; 59:257–262.

11   Rao TL, Jacobs KH, El-Etr AA. Reinfarction following anesthesia in patients with myocardial infarction. *Anesthesiology.* 1983; 59:499–505.

12   Freeman LN, Schachat AP, Manolio TA, Enger C. Multivariate analysis of factors associated with unplanned admission in 'outpatient' ophthalmic surgery. *Ophthalmic Surg.* 1988; 19:719–723.

13   Schein OD, Katz J, Bass EB, Tielsch JM, Lubomski LH, Feldman MA, Petty BG, Steinberg EP. The value of routine preoperative medical testing before cataract surgery. Study of Medical Testing for Cataract Surgery. *N Engl J Med.* 2000; 342:168–175.

14   Kraushar MF, Turner MF. Medical malpractice litigation in cataract surgery. *Arch Ophthalmol.* 1987; 105:1339–1343.

15   Lutner RE, Roizen MF, Stocking CB, Thisted RA, Kim S, Duke PC, Pompei P, Cassel CK. The automated interview versus the personal interview. Do patient responses to preoperative health questions differ? *Anesthesiology.* 1991; 75:394–400.

16   Roizen MF. More preoperative assessment by physicians and less by laboratory tests. *N Engl J Med.* 2000; 342:204–205.

17   Kost GJ. Critical limits for urgent clinician notification at US medical centers. *JAMA.* 1990; 263:704–707.

18   Duker JS, Belmont JB, Benson WE, Brooks HL Jr, Brown GC, Federman JL, Fischer DH, Tasman WS. Inadvertent globe perforation during retrobulbar and peribulbar anesthesia. Patient characteristics, surgical management, and visual outcome. *Ophthalmology.* 1991; 98:519–526.

19   Speaker MG, Guerriero PN, Met JA, Coad CT, Berger A, Marmor M. A case-control study of risk factors for intraoperative suprachoroidal expulsive hemorrhage. *Ophthalmology.* 1991; 98:202–209.

20   Tabandeh H, Sullivan PM, Smahliuk P, Flynn HW Jr, Schiffman J. Suprachoroidal hemorrhage during pars plana vitrectomy. Risk factors and outcomes. *Ophthalmology.* 1999; 106:236–42.

21   Eagle KA, Brundage BH, Chaitman BR, Ewy GA, Fleisher LA, Hertzer NR, Leppo JA, Ryan T, Schlant RC, Spencer WH 3rd, Spittell JA Jr, Twiss RD, Ritchie JL, Cheitlin MD, Gardner TJ, Garson A Jr, Lewis RP, Gibbons RJ, O'Rourke RA, Ryan TJ. Guidelines for perioperative cardiovascular evaluation for noncardiac surgery. Report of the American College of Cardiology/American Heart Association Task Force on Practice Guidelines. Committee on Perioperative Cardiovascular Evaluation for Noncardiac Surgery. *Circulation.* 1996; 93:1278–1317.

22   Campeau L. Letter: Grading of angina pectoris. *Circulation.* 1976; 54:522–523.

23   Dajani AS, Taubert KA, Wilson W, Bolger AF, Bayer A, Ferrieri P, Gewitz MH, Shulman ST, Nouri S, Newburger JW, Hutto C, Pallasch TJ, Gage TW, Levison ME, Peter G, Zuccaro G Jr. Prevention of bacterial endocarditis. Recommendations by the American Heart Association. *Circulation.* 1997; 96:358–366.

24   The sixth report of the Joint National Committee on prevention, detection, evaluation, and treatment of high blood pressure. *Arch Intern Med.* 1997; 157:2413–2446.

25   Smetana GW. Preoperative pulmonary evaluation. *N Engl J Med.* 1999; 340:937–44.

26   Schade DS. Surgery and diabetes. *Med Clin North Am.* 1988; 72:1531–1543.

27   Burgos LG, Ebert TJ, Asiddao C, Turner LA, Pattison CZ, Wang-Cheng R, Kampine JP. Increased intraoperative cardiovascular morbidity in diabetics with autonomic neuropathy. *Anesthesiology.* 1989; 70:591–597.

28   Salem M, Tainsh RE Jr, Bromberg J, Loriaux DL, Chernow B. Perioperative gluco-corticoid coverage. A reassessment 42 years after emergence of a problem. *Ann Surg.* 1994; 219:416–425.

29   Kearon C. Perioperative management of long-term anticoagulation. *Semin Thromb Hemost.* 1998; 24 Suppl 1:77–83.

30   Langston RH. What is the risk of complications from cataract surgery in patients taking anticoagulants? *Cleve Clin J Med.* 2001; 68:97–98.

6

Orbital Regional Anaesthesia

Dr Chandra M. Kumar
Dr Gary L. Fanning

Introduction

With the introduction of topical anaesthesia for cataract surgery, some predicted that injection techniques for ocular anaesthesia would become much less important. This certainly has been true for many cataract surgeons, but not all. According to Leaming[1], 53% of respondents to the ASCRS annual survey used either a retrobulbar or peribulbar technique for anaesthesia in cataract surgery. This indicates that a number of surgeons still prefer a regional block over topical anaesthesia for some or all of their patients.

Although numerically the most significant, cataract extraction is not the only procedure performed on the eye. Strabismus surgery, retinal surgery, panretinal photocoagulation, and other major eye procedures are carried out under general or regional anaesthesia, although topical anaesthesia has been described for use in strabismus surgery[2] and others. In addition, many feel strongly that certain patients are relatively poor candidates for topical anaesthesia for cataract surgery.[3] It seems unlikely, therefore, that regional anaesthesia of the orbit will completely disappear from ophthalmic surgical practice.

The purpose of this chapter is to review and describe techniques for performing orbital regional anaesthesia. Whilst we will refer to anatomy and complications in this chapter, the reader is encouraged to study Chapters 2 and 14, which are devoted to those subjects.

Terminology

Retrobulbar Block
The classic description of a retrobulbar block was provided by Atkinson.[4] In this technique a long (1½") needle is inserted in the orbit into the intraconal space behind

the globe. As the needle tip lies well back toward the apex of the orbit near where the sensory nerves exit and motor nerves enter, only small volumes (1.5–4 ml) of local anaesthetic are required to achieve anaesthesia. If orbicularis oculi anaesthesia is required, one must perform a separate facial nerve block when using this deep, low-volume technique.

Peribulbar (Parabulbar, Peri-orbital, Peri-ocular, Extraconal) Block
In this block, no attempt is made to enter the intraconal space with the needle, and shorter (½–1") needles are used. Because the needle tip is further away from the apex, one must depend on diffusion of the anaesthetic within the orbit to reach the orbital nerves. As a result, larger volumes (6–10 ml) of anaesthetic are injected to achieve satisfactory results. There are a number of variations of this type of block.

Sub-Tenon's Block
In sub-Tenon's block, Tenon's capsule is elevated from the sclera, and local anaesthetic is infused into the sub-Tenon's/episcleral space resulting in anaesthesia and akinesia.

Controversy in Nomenclature

Problems exist regarding the terminology used in describing orbital regional anaesthesia. For example, not everyone agrees on the meaning of the term intraconal. Some consider the cone to be that area of the orbit near the apex where the bellies of the extraocular muscles are relatively large and very close together. In the opinion of others the intraconal space incorporates all the area behind the globe within the borders of the tendons and bellies of the rectus muscles. These proponents further divide the intraconal space into a shallow (anterior) portion and a deep (posterior) portion. Many authors described a membrane, the intermuscular septum, which separated the intraconal and extraconal spaces. It is now well established and recognised by most that there is no true intermuscular septum that defines the border between the intra and extraconal spaces. Ripart et al.[5] recently demonstrated clearly that solutions easily diffuse into the intraconal space when injected into the extraconal space and vice versa. Still others argue about the term retrobulbar, pointing out correctly that any needle longer than about 5/8" will be retrobulbar when fully inserted into the orbit. These proponents would prefer to use the terms intraconal and extraconal (or periconal) for describing a block. Another aspect of the ongoing discussion about these terms is the difference in practices. Many practitioners use a single-shot block technique, whilst others prefer to inject in two separate areas. This has led to the terms combined retro/peribulbar block, combined intra/extraconal block, or simply combined block. In this chapter the term orbital regional anaesthesia will be used when discussing orbital block techniques in general.

Anatomical Considerations

Prior to performing any regional anaesthetic, thorough knowledge of the anatomical relationships of the area is essential. Nowhere is this more important than in the orbit, where many delicate structures are packed into a 30-ml space. The average globe (23.5 mm axial length) will occupy approximately 7 ml of the orbit, the remainder being filled with fat, extraocular muscles, vascular structures, nerves, lacrimal gland, and connective tissue.

The schematic drawings in this chapter were inspired by the descriptions of Dutton[6], Koornneef[7], and Ettl et al.[8] The reader is encouraged to refer to these works for more detailed anatomical information.

Figure 1 is a drawing of a frontal section of the orbit through the anterior portion of the globe perpendicular to the optic nerve, demonstrating where many of the

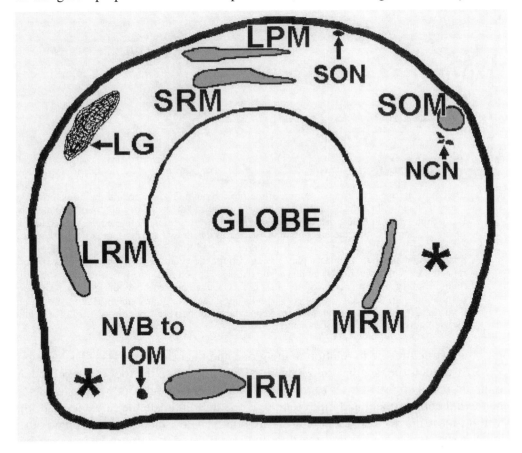

Fig. 1. This drawing of a frontal section through the right orbit shows the relationships of the important orbital structures in the anterior portion of the orbit. Note that the globe is slightly closer to the orbital roof than floor and to the lateral wall than to the medial. The asterisks indicate the fat-filled, relatively avascular, compartments that are the safest areas in which to insert needles into the orbit.

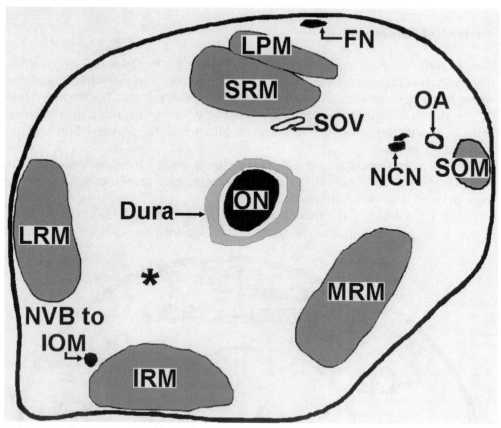

Fig. 2.   This drawing depicts a frontal section of the orbit about 5–10 mm behind the hind surface of
the eye. Note the location of the inferior rectus muscle and the neurovascular bundle to the inferior oblique muscle. These structures are in great danger of injury from needles placed too far
medially. Note also that there is only one asterisk in this drawing. This spot is where the tip of
a 1–1¼" inch needle should end up if properly inserted into the corner of the inferotemporal
quadrant and aimed to intersect a plane going through the lateral limbus. The superonasal quadrant is filled with many important and easily damaged structures: superior oblique muscle, ophthalmic artery, end branches of the nasociliary nerve, and the beginning of the superior
ophthalmic vein. The large optic nerve with its dural sheath is quite evident. Having the patient
hold the eye in neutral or lateral gaze keeps the optic nerve away from the tip of a needle
inserted into the inferotemporal quadrant.

important structures lie in relation to the globe and the orbital margins. The drawing
correctly reflects the fact that the globe lies slightly closer to the roof of the orbit than
to the floor and slightly closer to the lateral wall than to the medial. The asterisks in
the medial compartment and inferotemporal quadrant indicate the safest areas of the
orbit for inserting needles, as these areas are relatively avascular and contain no other
delicate structures. Notice that the inferotemporal asterisk is more lateral than has
been classically described. Most authors describe inserting the inferotemporal needle at the junction of the lateral third and medial two-thirds of the lower lid. This
point is far too medial and puts the following structures at risk of damage from the
needle: the inferior oblique muscle, the neurovascular bundle to the inferior oblique

muscle, and the inferior rectus muscle. Figure 2 is a similar frontal section approximately 5–10 mm behind the hind surface of the eye. It is unnecessary to place a needle, either intraconally or extraconally, any deeper than this in order to achieve adequate orbital anaesthesia. One notices in this drawing that a number of important structures are found in the superonasal quadrant.

Although still preferred by some, the superonasal quadrant is a dangerous place to insert needles. One finds there the trochlea, the tendon and belly of the superior oblique muscle, the ophthalmic artery, branches of the nasociliary nerve, and the origin of the superior ophthalmic vein. Figure 3 is a picture of an orbital dissection, showing how vulnerable the ophthalmic artery and other structures are in the superonasal quadrant. Use of the superonasal quadrant should be discouraged.

Figure 4, which is 15–20 mm behind the hind surface of the globe, illustrates why placing a needle far back in the orbit is dangerous. In this area the bellies of the extraocular muscles are large and close together. Everything here is packed tightly, giving rise to the term 'pickle jar' when referring to this part of the orbit. One can readily spear a pickle in a full jar in which the pickles are packed closely together, just as the bellies of the rectus muscles are in the posterior orbit. Nerves and vessels,

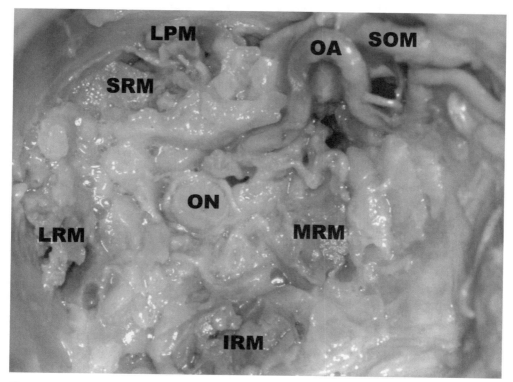

Fig. 3. This picture of an orbital dissection at about the level of Figure 2 shows how large and tortuous the ophthalmic artery can be in the superonasal quadrant as it courses along the belly of the superior oblique muscle. Injection of anaesthetic into the this artery has two unwanted consequences: the almost instantaneous onset of a grand mal seizure and an arterial retrobulbar haemorrhage.

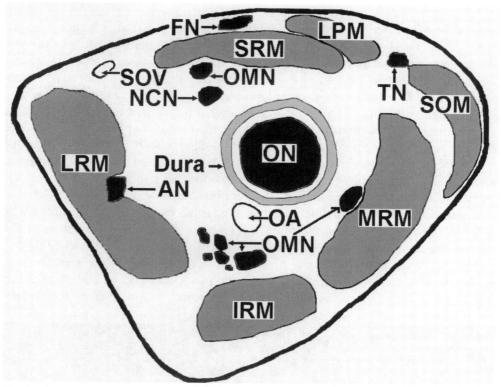

Fig. 4. A section 15–20 mm behind the hind surface of the eye leaves little doubt as to how dangerous it is to put needles so deeply into the orbit. The nerves, blood vessels, and muscle bellies are quite large and are held closely together in this area of the orbit near the apex. This makes penetrating them quite easy, just as easy as spearing a pickle in a full pickle jar.

which are quite large and enter the rectus muscles at the junctions of their middle and posterior thirds, may be injured by needles placed deeply. Intramuscular injection is an additional potential complication. Damage to the nerves, vessels, and/or muscles may lead to permanent strabismus. Being held tightly by the extraocular muscles near the orbital apex, the optic nerve is at risk of being damaged by needles placed so deeply. The needle tip may enter the extension of the subarachnoid space surrounding the optic nerve. Injection into this space results in brainstem anaesthesia, a potentially fatal complication of orbital regional anaesthesia.

The fascial sheath (Tenon's capsule) is a dense fibrous layer of elastic connective tissue surrounding the globe and extraocular muscles in the anterior orbit (Figure 5).[9] It originates at the limbus, extends posteriorly to the optic nerve, and blends with the connective tissue sheaths of the extraocular muscles. The penetration of Tenon's capsule by the rectus muscles divides the capsule into anterior and posterior portions. Anteriorly Tenon's capsule is adherent to the sclera for about 1.5 mm from the limbus. Because the conjunctiva remains fused with Tenon's capsule, the sub-Tenon's space can be directly accessed through an incision 2 to 3 mm from the limbus. The posterior part of the Tenon's capsule passes around to the optic nerve, separating the

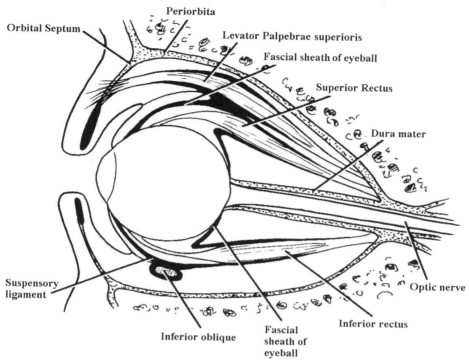

Fig. 5. Anatomical sketch of the orbit showing Tenon's capsule (reproduced with permission from Blackwell Scientific Publication Ltd).

globe from the contents of the retrobulbar space. The sheath fuses with the dura surrounding the optic nerve and with the sclera where the nerve enters the globe. Tenon's capsule is pierced by the ciliary nerves and vessels and by the vortex veins.

Preparation of the Patient

Prior to performing an orbital block, one should carefully evaluate the patient (see Chapter 5). Review of the medical history and physical examination is important. The patient's current medications, compliance, and known drug allergies should be noted. Hopefully the patient will have been advised to continue taking all routine medications, especially antihypertensives. Patients taking warfarin compounds may remain on them for cataract surgery as long as a recent prothrombin time is in the therapeutic range (INR of 2–3).[10–15] Taking patients off warfarin is unnecessary for uncomplicated cataract surgery and poses risks of thrombotic or embolic phenomena. For more complicated procedures, such as enucleation, retinal surgery, or tumour surgery, it may be appropriate to discontinue warfarin after consulting with the patient's physician.

A thorough external examination of both eyes should be performed to rule out any acute infectious process, such as conjunctivitis or chalazion. Abnormalities of extraocular motor functions should also be noted and recorded. The operative side should be confirmed both by examination of the record and questioning of the patient.

Knowing the length of the eye is important, because eyes longer than 26 mm in axial length are at greater risk of perforation.[16–19] For patients undergoing cataract surgery, measurement of the axial length of the eye is always done as part of the calculation for the intraocular lens. The axial length should be noted in the anaesthetic record. This often requires asking the surgeon to supply this information in the preoperative note or in the preoperative orders. For patients not having cataract surgery, it is wise to look at the eyeglass prescription, if this is available. Patients with long eyes will have spherical equivalents of –3.00 to –12 dioptres or greater. If their eyeglass prescriptions are not available, simply ask the patients if they need glasses to read or to see far away. Those needing glasses to see far away and who have needed them to do so since childhood are myopic and may have long eyes.

The relationship between the globe and the orbit is crucial. It is important to know if one is dealing with a large or small orbit and to assess how the globe is situated within the orbit. Is it a large or small globe? Is the globe deeply seated within the orbit or is it proptotic? A large globe deeply seated in a tight orbit may preclude safe needle techniques, and other techniques, such as sub-Tenon's block, topical anaesthesia, or general anaesthesia, might be better advised. It is essential for each practitioner to make this judgement before proceeding with an orbital block.

One must also determine whether or not the patient has had prior ophthalmic surgery or orbital trauma. Scleral buckling procedures tend to elongate the eye and may also result in significant scarring within the orbit. This is particularly important if sub-Tenon's anaesthesia is planned, as scleral perforation has been reported in a patient with a previous scleral buckling procedure.[20] Prior orbital trauma may result in disfiguration or scarring that would render orbital regional anaesthesia unsafe. The same may be said of other orbital abnormalities, such as the presence of a tumour or a vascular abnormality like a giant haemangioma. Advanced stages of dysthyroid orbitopathy may also preclude safe needle techniques, because the bellies of the rectus muscles become enormous, making them especially vulnerable to injury from needles.

Prior to performing a block, the patient should be properly monitored, preferably using an ECG, non-invasive blood pressure, and pulse oximetry. Supplemental oxygen should also be given, particularly when sedation is used. An intravenous cannula with a self-sealing injection port should be in place. In addition to being a useful route for administering sedation, it is also essential should a critical event occur. The administration of intravenous fluids is not routinely indicated for cataract surgery and other brief ophthalmic procedures.

Control of blood pressure is controversial. Some practitioners defer surgery if systolic pressures are elevated to levels of 200 mm Hg or more. Although it is very difficult to find evidence in the literature to support them, others feel strongly that it is important to maintain systolic pressures below the 150–170 mm Hg range both before performing an orbital block and during surgery. The reasons for tight control are to reduce cardiac stress; to reduce the incidence of intraoperative vascular complications, such as expulsive haemorrhage; and to minimize the consequences of retrobulbar haemorrhage secondary to the orbital block. If one chooses to treat elevated blood pressures, there are several options available. Often small amounts of anxiolytic agents, such as midazolam, will help to control modest elevations. Intravenous labetalol (10–20 mg) is useful if the patient shows signs of apprehension, tachycardia, or unresponsiveness to anxiolytics and has no contraindications to beta-blocking drugs. Calcium-channel blocking drugs, such as oral nifedipine (5 mg mixed in 120 ml of water) or intravenous nicardipine (0.5–1.0 mg), are also effective and are useful in patients with absolute or relative contraindications to beta-blocking drugs. Care must be taken in acutely lowering blood pressure in patients with known aortic stenosis, coronary artery disease, cerebrovascular disease, and/or renovascular disease.

Some practitioners sedate their patients heavily before performing orbital regional anaesthesia, others find that this is unnecessary and feel that deep sedation for this block is dangerous. One can perform this block comfortably for the patient using modest amounts of sedation (1–2 mg midazolam combined with 25–50 mg of thiopentone or similar combinations) or no sedation at all by observing a few simple precautions. One may begin with a skin wheal of 0.1% lidocaine injected through a 30G needle. Painless injection can be achieved by using a short, sharp, fine-gauge needle; by warming anaesthetic solution to about 35°C; and by injecting slowly (no more than 1 ml every 15–20 seconds). If one takes these precautions and the patient experiences significant pain, it may indicate injection of anaesthetic solution into an inappropriate place (muscle, nerve, or sclera).

The use of a trained assistant is very helpful when performing orbital regional anaesthesia. In addition to helping hold the head still and the eyelid open, the assistant can watch the monitors, calm the patient, and assist the anaesthetist. The assistant is also able to ensure that the position of the patient's head is the same each time.

Needle Choices for Injection Techniques

A variety of needles are available for performing injection techniques. It is controversial as to which kind of needle should be employed.

Needle Length

Atkinson[4] described the use of a 1.38" (35 mm) 22G needle in performing an orbital block. One can reach the deepest portions of the orbit using a needle this long in many patients. In his paper, Atkinson argues that his technique minimized damage to nerves and vessels. However, Katsev et al.[21] measured the distance from the junction of the lateral third and medial two-thirds of the orbital rim to the optic canal in a series of cadavers. They assumed that any needle that could reach within 7 mm of the optic canal was relatively dangerous, as this is the area where structures are most densely packed. They suggested that any needle longer than 1¼" (32 mm) is potentially hazardous in

15–20% of patients. This is an important work that underscores the dangers of long needles. As many others have reported excellent results using 1¼" or shorter needles, *one should not use needles longer than 1¼" when performing injection techniques.*

Needle Gauge

Advocates of the larger gauge (22–25G) needle find that the stiffer needle allows better 'feel' during insertion. Those who prefer the fine needle (27–30G) argue that small gauge needles give better tactile information and are less likely to damage intraorbital structures. Grizzard et al.[22] reported that the ultimate visual results in globes perforated with fine-gauge needles are better than in those perforated with large. Additional arguments in favour of fine, sharp needles are that they are easier and much less painful to insert.

Needle Shape

There are several variations of curved needles used for orbital blocks. The Straus needle[23,24] incorporates a curved section with a straight section. Using this needle, one inserts at the inferotemporal corner and allows the curve of the needle to skirt the globe so that the tip ends up in the retrobulbar area. Straus reported excellent results in 40,000 patients using this needle. Curved needles have also been described by Teichmann and Uthoff.[25] In their technique a curved needle is introduced inferiorly in the midline, again allowing the curve to skirt the globe in order to place the tip in the retrobulbar, intraconal area. Although they reported great success in 20,000 patients using this needle, one cannot advocate purposely putting needles through the inferior rectus muscle as they described. They did not report the incidence of postoperative diplopia in their paper, stating only that none of their patients 'had trauma to the inferior rectus or inferior oblique that resulted in clinically appreciable sequelae.' Hamilton et al.[26] has described putting a 10° bend half way along the shaft of a 27G straight needle and inserting it through the inferotemporal corner, arguing that the bend helps to keep the tip of the needle away from the globe initially and then ensures that it ends up in the intraconal space behind the globe (Dr Hamilton has now abandoned the bent needle technique – personal communication).

Straight needles have long been used in performing orbital blocks. One advantage of the straight needle is its simplicity of use. An additional advantage is the lower cost of straight needles compared with commercially produced curved needles. To date the evidence is not convincing that curved needles are either safer or more effective than straight.

Needle Tip

The sharp versus dull controversy continues. Advocates of dull needles, such as Waller et al.,[27] claim that they are less likely to perforate the globe, owing to greater force being required. Any needle capable of penetrating the unbroken skin is able to perforate the globe. Advocates of fine, sharp needles point to the ease of their insertion, better tactile information, less pain compared with dull needles, and the possibility of less damage than with dull needles should one be so unfortunate as to perforate the globe. In order for a dull needle to be substantially safer than a sharp one, it has to be very dull and of large gauge. These needles are hard to get through the skin and result in more pain on insertion than do fine, sharp needles, requiring deeper sedation. The argument that one can feel a dull needle 'popping' into the cone is specious, because there is no clearly defined intermuscular septum. A 'popping' sensation can occur when traversing a connective tissue septum, but it can also occur when entering a vessel, a nerve, the dura, a muscle, or the sclera. It is also unfounded that dull needles are especially indicated in patients with long eyes.[27] In fact, these patients often have exceptionally thin sclera that is readily perforated by even a very dull needle.

Techniques

Classic Retrobulbar Block

Credit for the classical retrobulbar block is given to Atkinson.[4] Confusion exists between Atkinson's original description and the illustration, which accompanied it. He described the point of entry as the 'inferior temporal margin of the orbit.' The illustration appears to show the needle entering the orbit at about the junction of the lateral third and medial two-thirds of the inferior orbital rim. As a result, most people have been taught that the Atkinson block described the needle being inserted into the inferotemporal quadrant of the orbit at this point. The patient was directed to gaze upward and inward. This position should not be used, as it brings the macula and optic nerve directly into the path of the needle. Atkinson advocated this position in order to move the anterior fascial elements connecting the rectus muscles out of the way of the needle tip during insertion. Modern authors advise the patient's gaze to be in the neutral position during insertion of the needle. Aimed at the orbital apex and inserted fully, the needle tip ends up deeply placed in many orbits. Injection of 1.5–4 ml of anaesthetic solution results in excellent orbital anaesthesia and akinesia. It does not, however, result in akinesia of the orbicularis oculi muscle, so that a separate facial nerve block needs to be performed if total lid akinesia and absence of 'squeezing' is desired. Although commonly used in the past and still practiced extensively today, this block and all deep orbital blocks are attended by an undesirably high incidence of certain complications, including retrobulbar haematoma, optic nerve damage, brainstem anaesthesia, and extraocular muscle dysfunction, as would be predicted from knowing the anatomy of the orbit. The fact that most practitioners of this block use a needle longer than Atkinson did (1.5" instead of 1.38") adds to the danger of this block.

Peribulbar Blocks

Numerous forms of peribulbar, periocular, or extraconal anaesthesia have been described and are being practiced since first reported by Davis and Mandel[28] in 1986. Most have in common the use of a short needle (⅝–1¼") and insertion of the needle into the extraconal space. These blocks require a larger volume of local anaesthetic

(6–10 ml) in order to achieve the same degree of orbital anaesthesia and extraocular muscle akinesia as the Atkinson type, because they rely on diffusion of anaesthetic solution into the intraconal space. A benefit of these larger volumes is that sufficient anaesthetic flows retrograde through the orbital septum to produce akinesia of the orbicularis oculi, so that a separate facial nerve block is usually unnecessary.

Davis and Mandel[28] described a two-injection technique using a 1¼" needle in which an inferior extraconal injection was followed by a superior extraconal injection. Their illustration shows the needles entering quite close to the midpoints of the inferior and superior orbital rims. With both injections, no attempt was made to place the needle within the cone. A total of about 6–8 ml of anaesthetic was used, some of it being deposited superficially under the orbicularis oculi. They stated that when learning this technique anaesthesia was incomplete about 50% of the time. After gaining experience, additional injections were needed in about 10% of patients. Orbicularis oculi akinesia was sufficient to allow them to omit a separate facial nerve block, as is true with most high-volume, peribulbar techniques. Amaurosis, a common finding in intraconal blocks, did not occur in their patients, but they did not find this to be a problem. Davis and Mandel stressed the safety of peribulbar anaesthesia in this initial report, and their impression was later confirmed by a multicentre study of over 16,000 patients that they published in 1994.[29]

Bloomberg[30] described his technique as anterior periocular anaesthesia. Using a 1" 27G needle, he inserted it at the junction of the lateral third and medial two thirds of the lower lid, aiming toward the floor of the orbit to stay away from the conal space. The needle was advanced only about ¾", not to the hub. He slowly injected local anaesthetic until 8–10 ml had been injected, less if the globe started to become tense. His rate of re-block (i.e., supplementation) was approximately 10% if he desired complete akinesia.

Ripart et al.[31] described a periocular injection in which a 25G short-bevelled needle is inserted into the semilunar fold between the globe and caruncle. The needle is directed medially, the globe rotating medially along with it. The needle is slowly brought to an antero-posterior position until a 'click' is felt as the needle passes through the medial check ligament into the extraconal space medial to the medial rectus muscle. The globe generally returns spontaneously to primary gaze after feeling this 'click.' At this point a total of 8–10ml of anaesthetic is injected. He reported that his group achieved a supplementation rate less than 5% after gaining experience with this technique.

Hustead et al.[32] earlier described a similar medial pericone block. In their technique the fat-filled compartment medial to the medial rectus muscle is entered medial to the caruncle using a ½" needle. A variation of their technique is more fully described below.

Combined Retro/Peribulbar Block
In this block, which has a number of varieties and advocates,[33] two injections are routinely made, one intraconal and one extraconal. In this description, the anaesthetist is

standing on the ipsilateral side of the patient, although in practice some prefer to stand at the head of the patient or rarely on the contralateral side. The first (intraconal) injection is made at the inferotemporal corner of the orbit. The point of insertion is approximately 1–1½ cm below the lateral canthus. It is essential to keep to the extreme inferotemporal corner, not to the more medial point as has been taught in the past. (Figure 6) In patients with especially short palpebral fissures, the insertion point is actually lateral to the lateral canthus. The corner of the orbit, where one often feels a small notch, is located by palpation, and a skin wheal is raised at this point using dilute (0.1%) lidocaine solution. Some anaesthetists prefer to use the transconjunctival approach after applying topical anaesthetic, which is acceptable. The transcutaneous approach is definitely easier in patients with short palpebral fissures and in those who are very sensitive and protective. With the patient's head in neutral position and with the eyes in primary gaze, a 1–1¼" (25–32 mm) sharp 27G needle is inserted. The bevel of the needle should be facing the globe so to keep the tip away from the sclera. A variation of the technique used by one of the authors (GF) has the bevel facing the globe at the beginning of insertion until the tip is well beyond the equator of the globe, after which the needle is spun 180° to help guide the tip toward the intraconal space and away from the orbital wall. The needle is directed along the diagonal of the orbit

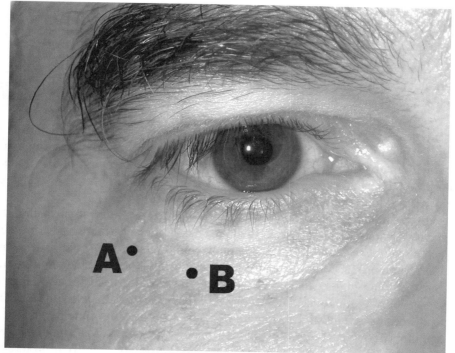

Fig. 6.   Point A indicates the inferotemporal corner of the orbit where a small notch can often be felt. This is the preferred location for inserting a needle into the inferotemporal quadrant of the orbit. Point B is the junction of the lateral third and medial two-thirds of the orbital rim, the point classically recommended for this injection.

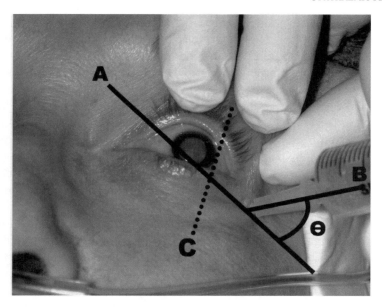

Fig. 7. Line A represents the inferotemporal to superonasal diagonal of the orbit. The syringe and needle should be aligned along this line. Dotted line C represents a sagittal plane going through the
lateral limbus. Line B is a straight line along the shaft of the needle and barrel of the syringe.
The needle is inserted posteromedially through the skin (or conjunctiva) on line A so that the tip
of the needle will intersect plane C just behind the hind surface of the eye. Angle θ will be different in every patient. In the average patient it is about 45°. If the eye is short and/or proptotic
the angle will be less than 45°; and if it is long and/or deeply set, the angle will be greater than
45°.

(inferotemporal to superonasal) (Figure 7) and is aimed posteromedially behind to
intersect a plane going through the lateral limbus at a point 5–10 mm behind the hind
surface of the globe. The needle should not be directed toward the orbital apex. The
postero-medial angle (angle θ in Figure 7) with the frontal plane will vary with each
patient, depending on the axial length of the eye and how deeply the globe is positioned within the orbit. In the average patient the angle will be close to 45°. In a short
and/or proptotic eye the angle will be relatively shallow or less than 45°, whilst in the
deeply set and long eye it will be much greater than 45°.

Insertion should be slow and deliberate with careful observation of the globe,
which should not move. If the globe starts to move, it may mean that the needle has
contacted sclera, and it should be immediately withdrawn. Initially the patient should
be maintaining primary gaze. Under no circumstances should the patient gaze medially, lest the optic nerve be delivered directly to the tip of the needle. One author (GF)
likes to have the patient gaze laterally toward the anaesthetist's nose after the tip of
the needle has passed the globe's equator. This protects both the optic nerve and macula, and globe movement by the patient reasonably assures one that the globe has not
been fixated by a perforating needle. Moving the eye slowly laterally is preferable to
the practice of some who move the needle back and forth ('stir the orbital contents')
to see if they have perforated the globe. The shoulder of the needle (where the hub
meets the shaft) should just touch the skin or be slightly short of it. The skin should

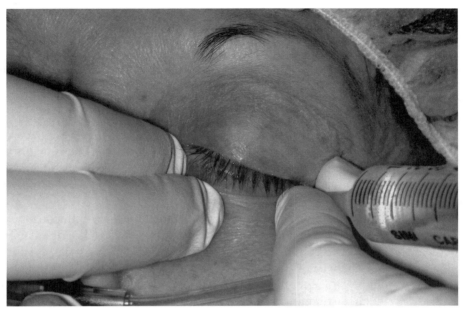

Fig. 8. The assistant is applying gentle pressure with two fingers over the medial half of the inferior orbital septum. The anaesthetist applies similar pressure over the lateral half whilst simultaneously holding firmly to the hub of the needle to prevent its being pushed too deeply into the orbit. Pressure over the inferior orbital septum during injection promotes flow of the injectate backwards and upwards instead of retrograde into the lower lid.

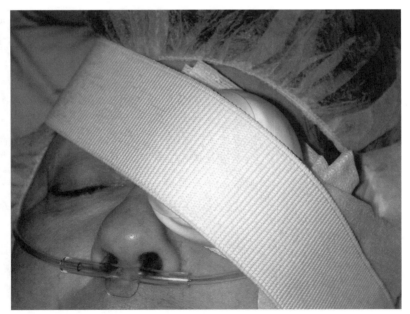

Fig. 9. After injection the eye is closed and covered with a dressing gauze and a compression device is applied. In the example seen here a soft, supple plastic ball is being used. Many prefer the Honan balloon. Care must be exercised to avoid excessive pressures (30 mm Hg or less) and excessive times (20 minutes or less).

not be indented because this may result in a 1¼" needle ending up as deeply in the orbit as a 1½" needle. After careful aspiration, anaesthetic solution is injected at the rate of 1 ml every 15–20 seconds. It is helpful to have the assistant place two fingers over the lower lid at the orbital margin in order to bolster the inferior orbital septum (Figure 8). Gentle pressure here encourages the injectate to flow posteriorly and superiorly instead of into the lower lid. During injection, the globe should be periodically palpated to ensure that it remains freely mobile within the orbit and does not become too tense. Normally 6–10 ml of solution can be easily injected, but occasionally only 4–5 ml can be injected without causing too much pressure within the orbit. On average 5–6 ml is required. After injection, an ocular compression device, such as a Honan balloon, is placed over the eye for five minutes (Figure 9).

After five minutes, the eye is examined for movement and the extraconal part of the block is performed. This is done in the medial canthal area, as described by Hustead et al.[32] A 27G 1" needle (Hustead et al. advocated a ½" 30G needle) is inserted into the little tunnel between the medial canthal fold and the caruncle (Figure 10). The needle should be aimed at the medial orbital wall and advanced carefully until the wall is just touched (Figure 11). The wall is extremely thin (lamina papyracea), so one must be especially cautious. After just touching the wall, the needle is withdrawn 1–2 mm and redirected to be inserted parallel to both the orbital wall and the

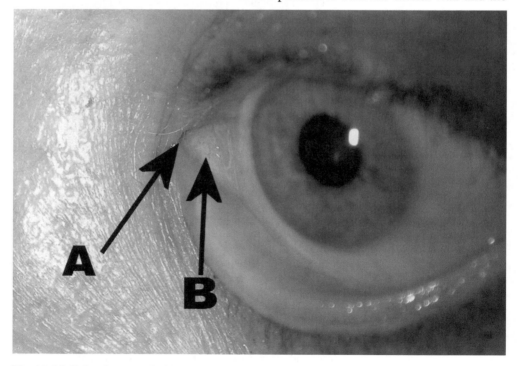

Fig. 10. Medial to the caruncle (Arrow B) and behind the medial canthus lies a small depression or tunnel (Arrow A). In performing the medial periconal injection, the 1" 27G needle is first inserted carefully into this little tunnel.

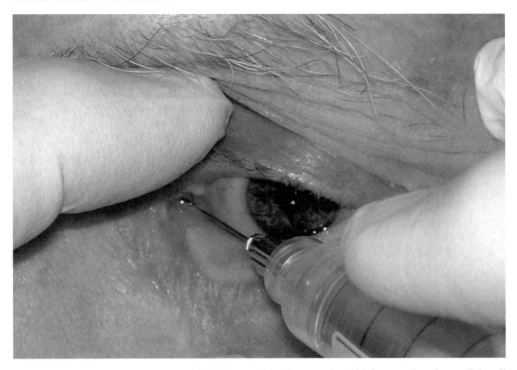

Fig. 11. The needle is slowly and carefully inserted into the tunnel until it just touches the medial wall of the orbit. The bone is incredibly thin in this area, so great care must be taken to avoid pushing the needle tip into the ethmoid sinus. After just touching bone, the needle is withdrawn about 1–2 mm and redirected to enter the orbit perpendicular to the frontal plane or just 5° medially.

orbital floor (i.e., 90° to the frontal plane), although Hustead et al. recommended angling about 5° medially in order to ensure missing the medial rectus muscle (Figure 12). The needle must be close to the wall but not subperiosteal. If the needle is not close to the wall and if it is inserted too deeply, injury to the medial rectus muscle can occur. During insertion the globe may briefly move medially as the needle goes through the medial check ligament. The 1" needle should be inserted until the shoulder lies no deeper than the plane of the iris. If one's needle is properly placed in the fatty compartment, it very nearly inserts itself in many patients because there is so little resistance. A needle longer than 1" should not be used, because the optic canal may be reached by a longer needle, endangering the optic nerve and/or ophthalmic artery.

After careful aspiration to rule out an intravascular location, one injects 2–4 ml of anaesthetic into this fat-filled compartment. Palpation of the globe is important during injection to prevent excessive intraorbital pressures. One may occasionally find a patient who can tolerate only 1–2 ml of anaesthetic agent in this compartment following the inferotemporal injection. On the other hand, some practitioners use only the medial canthal extraconal injection for orbital blocks and inject 8–10 ml of anaesthetic at this site.[30] Following this injection, the compression device is placed on the eye again and left in place for 10–20 minutes prior to surgery.

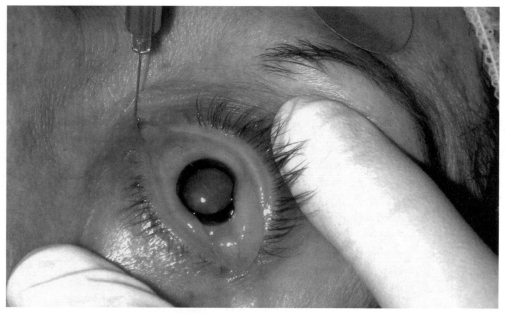

Fig. 12. The needle has now been redirected and is being inserted into the medial periconal, fat-filled compartment. In many patients there is so little resistance that the needle very nearly inserts itself. Under no circumstances should a needle longer than 1" be used, and the hub of the 1" needle should not go deeper than the plane of the iris.

Practitioners with adequate experience can achieve greater than 95% akinesia about 95% of the time with these two injections. In most patients the medial periconal injection is done to achieve complete akinesia of the medial rectus, superior oblique, and orbicularis oculi muscles, and it probably helps to prolong the block. It may be omitted if an adequate block results from the inferotemporal injection. If the inferotemporal injection produces a poor block, it usually means that it was injected extraconally. In this case it is often wise to repeat the inferotemporal injection if complete akinesia is desired. Some practitioners perform an extraconal injection in the superotemporal quadrant if the first two injections result in inadequate levator and/or superior rectus akinesia. If one chooses to do this rather than to repeat one of the other injections, it is important to remember that the superior half of the orbit contains the majority of the largest vessels, and care must be observed to prevent intravascular injection and retrobulbar haemorrhage.

Sub-Tenon's Block

The technique involves obtaining surface anaesthesia followed by dissection, insertion of a cannula, and subsequent administration of local anaesthetic agent into sub-Tenon's space. Sub-Tenon's anaesthesia is a modification of the original idea of Turnbull[34] and Swan.[35] Many modern descriptions have been reported.[36–42]

Surface Anaesthesia

Good surface anaesthesia is essential to providing a painless sub-Tenon's block. Amide and ester local anaesthetic drugs in appropriate concentrations are effective after topical application. Agents vary in their formulations and some contain preservatives and antibacterial substances.[43] Preservative-free preparations in single-dose containers are preferred.[43] All these agents may produce stinging on initial application. Surface anaesthesia can be achieved either by applying topical agents such as amethocaine (tetracaine), proxymetacaine (proparacaine) or benoxinate on the conjunctiva and cornea or by application of a sponge soaked with the topical agent in the area of dissection.

Access to sub-Tenon's Space

Access to sub-Tenon's space can be achieved from all four quadrants;[36,38,40,41] however, access to sub-Tenon's space by inferonasal quadrant dissection is the commonest approach described. Inferonasal quadrant placement of the cannula allows good fluid distribution superiorly whilst avoiding the area of surgery and reducing the risk of damage to the vortex veins. Fukasaku and Marron[40] advocate access through the superotemporal quadrant, whilst Ripart et al.[41] advocate access from the medial canthal side.

Surgical Dissection

Access to sub-Tenon's space is commonly obtained by surgical dissection but can be achieved by needle placement.[41] After obtaining initial pupillary dilatation and surface anaesthesia, the dissection is performed in the chosen quadrant. One author's preference (CMK) for access is the inferonasal quadrant as described by Stevens.[38] The lower lid is retracted either by an assistant or by placement of a lid speculum. The conjunctiva and Tenon's fascia are firmly gripped with non-toothed forceps 3–5 mm away from the limbus in the inferonasal quadrant and a small snip (1 to 2 mm) is made through the two layers with blunt-tipped, spring scissors. It is important to ensure that the cut includes both the conjunctiva and Tenon's capsule and that bare sclera is visible. The sub-Tenon's cannula, mounted on a syringe filled with local anaesthetic solution (2% lidocaine with 1:200,000 epinephrine and 5 units/ml hyaluronidase), is passed into sub-Tenon's space. The small volume of anaesthetic is injected intially to reduce pain and open up the space. The second injection is larger in volume and is introduced slowly. Some of the solution frequently appears in the subconjunctival space after injection, but this usually resolves with the application of gentle pressure.

In patients with previous detachment surgery, medial rectus surgery or pterygium surgery, insertion of the cannula through sub-Tenon's space may be difficult; therefore, dissection in another quadrant or another form of block is advisable.[44] Care is taken in performing a sub-Tenon's block in high myopes because of the occasional presence of a posterior staphyloma and /or scleral thinning.[44]

Cannula Choice

Various cannulae have been designed specifically for this technique. These can be either metal or plastic. Most metal cannulae are 1 inch long, are curved with a blunt end, and come in sizes from 19 to 23 gauge (Figure 13). The openings of these cannulae may be end holes or side holes. Greenbaum[39] invented a blunt 15G, D-shaped, flat bottomed, plastic cannula which is approximately 12 mm long and 2 mm in diameter. The opening on the flat bottom is designed so that it faces the sclera after insertion (Figure 14). Alternatives to these cannulae include: the Southampton cannula,[38] the ophthalmic irrigation cannula,[45] the intravenous cannula sheath,[42] and the Kumar–Dodds cannula (Figure 15).[46] The selection of a cannula depends on the availability and on the preference of the anaesthetist. Metal cannulae have been used most often in published studies. The placement of a polyethylene catheter into sub-Tenon's space has been described for surgery of long duration.[47]

Choice of Local Anaesthetic Agent

The ideal local anaesthetic agent for ophthalmic blocks should be non-toxic, painless to inject, and rapid in onset, producing dense motor and sensory blockade.[43] Its duration of action must be sufficiently long for surgery yet not excessively so. The speed of onset is partially determined by the properties of the agent but most importantly by its proximity to the nerves.[43] None of the present anaesthetic agents constitute the ideal. The choice of the currently available local anaesthetic agents depends on the personal preference of the anaesthetist. For sub-Tenon's block, lidocaine with or without epinephrine is the gold standard.

Volume of Local Anaesthetic

There is a wide variation in the volume of local anaesthetic used in sub-Tenon's block, and this has been a subject of debate. The volumes vary from 1 to 11 ml,[39,48] but 3 to 5 ml[38,49–51] is the usual range. Whilst small volumes may provide globe anaesthesia,[39] larger volumes are needed if akinesia is required.[51] Occasionally a repeat injection intraoperatively is required and is easily performed.

Complications and Problems

Sub-Tenon's anaesthesia has been associated with minor complications in the majority of reports. These include pain on injection, chemosis, conjunctival haemorrhage,

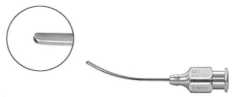

Fig. 13. Metal sub-Tenon cannula 19 G, 1 inch long, curved with blunt end (reproduced with permission from Katena Products Inc.).

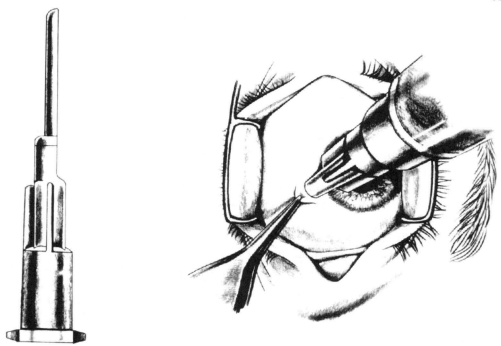

Fig. 14. Greenbaum plastic sub-Tenon cannula, 15G, 12 mm long, D-shaped with side opening (permission from Dr Scott Greenbaum[39]).

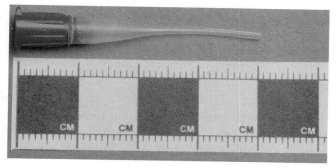

Fig. 15. Kumar–Dodds plastic cannula[46] 18 mm long.

short-lived muscle paresis,[52] and orbital haemorrhage.[53] Recently, scleral perforation during sub-Tenon's block has been reported in a patient who had previously undergone retinal surgery.[20]

Pain during Injection

Pain experienced during ophthalmic blocks can be multifactorial. The incidence of pain during sub-Tenon's injection is reported in up to 44% of patients,[38,45,50] and pain scores on a visual analogue scale (0=no pain, 10=worst imaginable) have been reported as high as 5.[38] Premedication or sedation of patients during sub-Tenon's injection has not added any benefit. Preoperative explanation of the procedure, good surface anaesthesia, gentle technique and reassurance is considered good practice and may reduce the discomfort and anxiety during the injection.

Chemosis

Chemosis signifies anterior injection of the anaesthetic agent. This usually occurs if a large volume of local anaesthetic is injected and if the Tenon's capsule is not dissected properly. The incidence of chemosis is as high as 25–40%[38,45,51] and is not confined to the site of injection. It resolves with digital pressure, and no intraoperative problems have been reported. Surgeons performing glaucoma surgery may feel that significant chemosis compromises the procedure.

Conjunctival Haemorrhage

Conjunctival haemorrhage can occur in a high proportion of cases and is almost inevitable following dissection. The incidence of haemorrhage varies from 20–100%.[38,45,50,51] This can be minimised by careful dissection avoiding damage to fine vessels plus the application of cautery and the use of topical epinephrine.[38,39] Patients are warned of the possibility of this occurrence preoperatively.

Loss of Local Anaesthetic Volume during Injection

Overspill of local anaesthetic during its administration is commonly observed.[38,50,51] This is likely to occur if the dissection is unsatisfactory, if injection meets resistance, if enlargement of the opening occurs during traction on the cannula or if large volumes are injected. Careful dissection and use of diathermy may minimise the loss.

Other Considerations

Ocular Compression

It is common to use some sort of compression device after an orbital injection. Occasionally this is simply done by gentle massage, but more often a ball or balloon is used.[54] Some authors contend that such compression is unwarranted or even dangerous.[55] Bowman et al.[56] measured changes in intraocular pressure (IOP) after peribulbar blocks with and without compression. In the group who received ocular compression after the block, the mean rise in IOP over pre-injection IOP was 11.44 mm Hg before compression. IOP fell to 2.42 mm Hg below the pre-injection pressure after 20 minutes of ocular compression. The group without compression experienced an initial rise of 9.45 mm Hg that fell only 2.42 mm Hg after 20 minutes.

It is useful to use some form of ocular compression after a high-volume orbital block in order to reduce IOP prior to intraocular surgery. This is particularly beneficial for cataract surgery, where increased vitreal pressure may severely compromise the procedure. For procedures such as strabismus surgery, compression is less important and may even be unwanted by the surgeon. In patients with known retinal circulatory insufficiency, ocular compression may be not be desirable. In cases of ocular trauma managed with an orbital regional anaesthetic, ocular compression must be avoided. If compression is used, it is important to ensure that the amount of pressure applied will not compromise intraocular circulation (30 mm Hg or less for a Honan balloon) and that the device not be left in place too long (i.e., more than about 20 minutes).

To date no studies have indicated that ocular compression is useful in sub-Tenon's block. If significant chemosis occurs after injection, digital compression may be all that is required.

Hyaluronidase

The addition of hyaluronidase to the local anaesthetic solution to improve its diffusion within the orbit after injection is a custom used by ophthalmic anaesthetists for a long time.[57] It is common to add 150 units of hyaluronidase to 5–10 ml of anaesthetic, for a final concentration of 15–30 units ml^{-1}. Atkinson described adding only 30 units of hyaluronidase to 5 mL of anaesthetic, a concentration of 6 units ml^{-1}. According to Robert Hustead, MD,[58] hyaluronidase was initially used clinically to improve the absorption of dermatoclysis solutions injected subcutaneously into the thigh. In those solutions 150 units of hyaluronidase were added to 1000 ml of fluid, and this was sufficient to allow very rapid absorption. Dr Hustead used only 0.5 units ml^{-1} for years in doing orbital regional anaesthesia and had excellent results. The concentration to use in the orbit lies somewhere between 0.5–15 units ml^{-1}.[59,60] (UK data sheet limits it to 15 iu ml^{-1}).

It is possible to achieve blocks in the orbit without using hyaluronidase. Bowman[61] described two groups of patients, one in which no hyaluronidase was used and another in which 150 units ml^{-1} was used. In this study there was no clinical difference between the two groups. In another study, Dempsey[62] compared three groups of patients with none, 50 units ml^{-1}, and 300 units ml^{-1} hyaluronidase in the anaesthetic mixture. The group receiving 300 units ml^{-1} had a slightly faster onset than the other two but otherwise was in no way different from the group receiving 50 units ml. Both hyaluronidase groups were only marginally different from those receiving none from the perspective of block quality.

Hyaluronidase helps the diffusion of the fluid mass within the orbit and may reduce the increased vitreal pressure resulting from a bolus of anaesthetic solution sitting behind the globe. If using a large-volume block technique, this is important, unless one allows a very long time with a compression device in place prior to surgery. During a recent shortage of hyaluronidase in the United States, several institutions reported an increased incidence of extraocular muscle dysfunction following the use of anaesthetic solutions without hyaluronidase.[63,64] There have been no randomised, double-blinded studies to confirm or deny these reports to date. It is a bit difficult to postulate how the lack of hyaluronidase leads to increased myotoxicity, but the possibility must be kept in mind.

Hyaluronidase improves the effectiveness and the quality of sub-Tenon's block block.[65,66]

Vasoconstrictors

Vasoconstrictors (epinephrine and felypressin) are commonly mixed with local anaesthetic solutions to increase the intensity and duration of block and to minimise bleeding from small vessels.[43] In addition, absorption of local anaesthetic is reduced thus avoiding a sudden surge in plasma levels. As epinephrine may cause vasoconstriction of the ophthalmic artery compromising the retinal circulation, the use of epinephrine containing solutions should be avoided in elderly patients suffering from cerebrovascular and cardiovascular diseases. If epinephrine is used, concentrations of 1:200,000 or less are recommended. Phacoemulsion cataract extraction is brief, and the duration of block achieved by lidocaine without epinephrine is usually sufficient.

pH Adjustment

Commercial preparations of lidocaine and bupivacaine are acidic, and the local anaesthetic exists predominantly in the charged ionic form.[43] It is only the non-ionised form of the agent that traverses the lipid membrane of the nerve to produce the conduction block. At higher pH values a greater proportion of local anaesthetic molecules exist in the non-ionised form, allowing more rapid influx into the neuronal cells. Alkalinisation has been shown to decrease the onset and prolong the duration of retrobulbar and peribulbar blocks.[67–69] Care must be taken in adjusting the pH of these solutions, because over-correction may cause precipitation of the anaesthetic agent.

Intraoperative Care

In the operating theatre patients should be placed comfortably on the table, being certain to pad them as necessary to assist their being able to lie still during surgery. Monitoring should continue as in the blocking area, with ECG, non-invasive blood pressure, and pulse oximetry. Nasal oxygen or some other form of increased air flow under the drapes should be provided in order to increase comfort, reduce the feeling of claustrophobia, and prevent carbon dioxide build up. The nurse or anaesthetist assigned to monitor the patient should hold the patient's hand, both to provide a feeling of reassurance and to provide a means of communication without talking. A squeeze of the hand by the patient signals the team that something is amiss and that surgery should be halted.

Controversy exists over whether or not a patient undergoing cataract extraction needs to be monitored in the operating theatre. In Denmark, for example, the majority of cataract extractions are done in the hospital and patients are not routinely monitored by an anaesthetist during surgery.[70] In Danish hospitals an anaesthetist is always free to respond to emergencies anywhere, including the eye room. In most other countries, monitoring of the patient in the operating theatre is routine. One report from a major teaching institution in the United States[71] measured the number of interventions required by the anaesthetist during cataract surgery. In their series of 560 patients, there were 186 patients (33%) who required at least one intervention from the anaesthetist. Those interventions included administration of cardiac and pulmonary drugs, management of blood glucose, administration of sedatives and analgesics, and others. They concluded that monitoring is important during this procedure.

The average cataract patient is an octogenarian with a variety of systemic illnesses. The most common of these are diabetes, hypertension, cardiovascular disease, cerebrovascular disease, and renovascular disease. Even fit-appearing patients can develop life-threatening problems in the operating theatre, making it difficult to predict who needs monitoring and who does not. Although rare, disastrous situations, including acute pulmonary oedema,[72] can occur either as a result of our interventions or simply by placing the patient supine with the feet up. Life-threatening but salvageable situations can occur in an elderly population due to chance alone. Arrhythmias, including ventricular tachycardia and fibrillation, arise with no forewarning. Coming into the theatre and being draped can be a frightening experience for many patients, resulting in hypertension, tachycardia, and a general feeling of doom. In summary, the purposes of monitoring the patient are to discover these problems early, to address them appropriately, to make the patient feel comfortable and safe, and to allow the surgeon to think about nothing but the proper operative care of the patient.

Abbreviations

AN = Abducens Nerve
FN = Frontal Nerve
IOM = Inferior Oblique Muscle
IRM = Inferior Rectus Muscle
LG = Lacrimal Gland
LPM = Levator Palpebrae Muscle
LRM = Lateral Rectus Muscle
MRM = Medial Rectus Muscle
NCN = Nasociliary Nerve

NVB = Neurovasular Bundle
OA = Ophthalmic Artery
OMN = Oculomotor Nerve
ON = Optic Nerve
SOM = Superior Oblique Muscle
SON = Supra Orbital Nerve
SOV = Superior Ophthalmic Vein
SRM = Superior Rectus Muscle
TN = Trochlear Nerve

References

1   Leaming DV. Special report: Practice styles and preferences of ASCRS members—2000 survey. *J Cataract Refract Surg.* 2001; 27:948–955.

2   Diamond GR. Topical anesthesia for strabismus surgery. *J Pediatr Ophthalmol Strabismus.* 1989; 26:86–90.

3   Fichman RA. Topical anesthesia. In: Davis DB, Mandel MR, editors. *Ophthalmology Clinics of North America,* vol. 11. 1998; 57–63.

4   Atkinson WS. Retrobulbar injection of anesthetic within the muscular cone. *Arch Ophthalmol.* 1936; 16:494–503.

5   Ripart J, Lefrant J, de la Coussaye J, Prat-Pradal D, Vivien B, Eledjam J. Peribulbar versus retrobulbar anesthesia for ophthalmic surgery. *Anesthesiology.* 2001; 94:56–62.

6   Dutton JJ. *Clinical and Surgical Orbital Anatomy.* WB Saunders Company, Philadelphia, 1994.

7   Koornneef L. Orbital septa: anatomy and function. *Ophthalmology.* 1979; 86:876–80.

8   Ettl A, Salomonowitz E, Koornneef L, Zonneveld FW. High-resolution MR imaging anatomy of the orbit. *Radiol Clin N Am*. 1998; 36:1021–1045.

9   Snell RS, Lemp MA, eds. *Clinical anatomy of the eye*. Blackwell Scientific Publications, Boston, 1989; 118–120.

10   McMahan LB. Anticoagulants and cataract surgery. *J Cataract Refract Surg*. 1988; 14:569–571.

11   Roberts CW, Woods SM, Turner LS. Cataract surgery in anticoagulated patients. *J Cataract Refract Surg*. 1991; 17:309–312.

12   McCormack P, Simcock PR, Tullo AB. Management of the anticoagulated patient for ophthalmic surgery. *Eye*. 1993; 7:749–750.

13   Saitoh AK, Saitoh A, Taniguchi H, Amemya T. Anticoagulation therapy and ocular surgery. *Ophthalmic Surg Lasers*. 1998; 29:909–915.

14   Kallio H, Paloheimo M, Maunuksela EL. Haemorrhage and risk factors associated with retrobulbar/peribulbar block: a prospective study in 1383 patients. *Br J Anaesth*. 2000; 85:708–711.

15   Morris A, Elder MJ. Warfarin therapy and cataract surgery. *Clin Experiment Ophthalmol*. 2000; 28:419–422.

16   Ramsay RC, Knobloch WH. Ocular perforation following retrobulbar anesthesia for retinal detachment surgery. *Am J Ophthalmol*. 1978; 86:61–64.

17   Duker JS, Belmont JB, Benson WE, Brooks HL Jr, Brown GC, Federman JL, Fischer DH, Tasman WS. Inadvertent globe perforation during retrobulbar and peribulbar anesthesia. Patient characteristics, surgical management, and visual outcome. *Ophthalmology*. 1991; 98:519–526.

18   Berglin L, Stenkula S, Algvere PV. Ocular perforation during retrobulbar and peribulbar injections. *Ophthalmic Surg Lasers*. 1995; 26:429–434.

19   Edge R, Navon S. Axial length and posterior staphyloma in Saudi Arabian cataract patients. *J Cataract Refract Surg*. 1999; 25:91–95.

20   Frieman BJ, Friedberg MA. Globe perforation associated with subtenon's anesthesia. *Am J Ophthalmol*. 2001; 131:520–521.

21   Katsev DA, Drews RC, Rose BT. An anatomic study of retrobulbar needle path length. *Ophthalmology*. 1989; 96:1221–1224.

22   Grizzard WS, Kirk NM, Pavan PR, Antworth MV, Hammer ME, Roseman RL. Perforating ocular injuries caused by anesthesia personnel. *Ophthalmology*. 1991; 98:1011–1016.

23   Straus JG. A new retrobulbar needle and injection technique. *Ophthalmic Surgery* 1988; 19:134–139.

24   Straus JG. Retrobulbar block: needle and technique. In: Davis DB, Mandel MR, editors. *Ophthalmology Clinics of North America*, vol. 11. 1998. pp 145–149.

25   Teichmann KD, Uthoff D. Retrobulbar (intraconal) anesthesia with a curved needle: technique and results. *J Cataract Refract Surg*. 1994; 20:54–60.

26   Hamilton RC. Gimbel Eye Centre technique of ocular regional anesthesia. In: Gills JP, Hustead RF, Sanders DR, editors. *Ophthalmic anesthesia*. Thorofare, New Jersey: Slack Incorporated, 1993; pp 134–40.

27   Waller SG, Taboada J, O'Connor P. Retrobulbar anesthesia risk: do sharp needles really perforate the eye more easily than blunt needles? *Ophthalmology*. 1993; 100:506–10.

28   Davis DB II, Mandel MR. Posterior peribulbar anesthesia: an alternative to retrobulbar anesthesia. *J Cataract Refract Surg*. 1986; 12:182–184.

29   Davis DB II, Mandel MR. Efficacy and complication rate of 16,224 consecutive peribulbar blocks: a prospective multicenter study. *J Cataract Refract Surg*. 1994; 20:327–337.

30   Bloomberg L. Anterior periocular anesthesia. In: Davis DB II, Mandel MR, editors. *Ophthalmology clinics of North America,* vol. 11. 1998; pp 47–56.

31   Ripart J, Lefrant J, Lalourcey L, Benbabaali M, Charavel P, Mainemer M, Prat-Pradal D, Dupeyron G, Eledjam J. Medial canthus (caruncle) single injection periocular anesthesia. *Anesth Analg.* 1996; 83:1234–38.

32   Hustead RF, Hamilton RC, Loken RG. Periocular local anesthesia: Medial orbital as an alternative to superior nasal injection. *J Cataract Refract Surg.* 1994; 20:197–201.

33   Hamilton RC. Retrobulbar block revisited and revised. *J Cataract Refract Surg.* 1996; 22:1147–1150.

34   Turnbull CS. *Med Surg Rep.* 1884; 29:628.

35   Swan KC. New drugs and techniques for ocular anesthesia. *Tr Am Acad Ophthalmol Otolaryngol.* 1956; 60:368.

36   Mein CE, Woodcock MG. Local anesthesia for vitreoretinal surgery. *Retina.* 1990; 10:47–49.

37   Hansen E, Mein C, Mazzoli R. Ocular anaesthesia for cataract surgery: A direct sub-Tenon's approach. *Ophth Surg.* 1990; 21:696–699.

38   Stevens JD. A new local anesthesia technique for cataract extraction by one quadrant sub-Tenon's infiltration. *Br J Ophthalmol.* 1992; 76:670–674.

39   Greenbaum S. Parabulbar anesthesia. *Am J Ophthalmol.* 1992; 114:776.

40   Fukasaku H, Marron JA. Sub-Tenon's pinpoint anesthesia. *J Cataract Refract Surg.* 1994; 20:468–471.

41   Ripart J, Metge L, Prat-Pradal D, Lopez FM, Eledjam JJ. Medial canthus single-injection episcleral (sub-tenon anesthesia): computed tomography imaging. *Anesth Analg.* 1998; 87:42–45.

42   Kumar CM, Williamson S, Chabria R. A simple method of sub-Tenon anaesthesia delivery. *Anaesthesia.* 2000; 55:612–613.

43   McLure HA. Rubin AP. Local anaesthesia for ophthalmic surgery. *Curr Anaesth Crit Care.* 1999; 10:40–47.

44   Guise PA. Single quadrant sub-Tenon's block. Evaluation of a new local anaesthetic technique for eye surgery. *Anaesth Intensive Care.* 1996; 24:241–244.

45   Verghese I, Sivraj P, Lai YK. The effectiveness of sub-Tenon's infiltration of local anaesthesia for cataract surgery. *Aust N Z J Ophthalmol.* 1996; 24:117–120.

46   Kumar CM, Dodds C. A disposable plastic sub-Tenon cannula. *Anaesthesia.* 2001; 56:399–400.

47   Behndig A. Sub-Tenon's anesthesia with a retained catheter in ocular surgery of longer duration. *J Cataract Refract Surg.* 1998; 24:1307–1309.

48   Li HK, Abouleish A, Grady J, Groeschel W, Gill KS. Sub-Tenon's injection for local anesthesia in posterior segment surgery. *Ophthalmology.* 2000; 107:41–46.

49   Tokuda Y, Oshika T, Amano S, Yoshitomi F, Inouye J. Anesthetic dose and analgesic effects of sub-Tenon's anesthesia. *J Cataract Ref Tract Surg.* 1999; 25:1250–1253.

50   Roman SJ, Chong Sit DA, Boureau CM, Auclin FX, Ullern MM. Sub-Tenon's anaesthesia: an efficient and safe technique. *Br J Ophthalmol.* 1997; 81:673–676.

51   Kumar CM, Dodds C. Evaluation of the Greenbaum sub-Tenon's block. *Br J Anaesth.* 2001; 87:631–633.

52   Spierer A, Schwalb E. Superior oblique muscle paresis after sub-Tenon's anesthesia for cataract surgery. *J Cataract Refract Surg.* 1999; 25:144–145.

53   Olitsky SE, Juneja RG. Orbital haemorrhage after the administration of sub-Tenon's infusion anaesthesia. *Ophthalmic Surg Lasers.* 1997; 28:145–146.

54   Quist LH, Stapleton SS, McPherson SD Jr. Preoperative use of the Honan intraocular pressure reducer. *Am J Ophthalmol.* 1983; 95:536–538.

55   Ellis J. Intraocular pressure changes after peribulbar injections with and without ocular compression (letter). *Br J Ophthalmol.* 1997; 81:421.

56   Bowman R, Liu C, Sarkies N. Intraocular pressure changes after peribulbar injections with and without ocular compression. *Br J Ophthalmol.* 1996; 80:394–397.

57   Atkinson WS. Use of hyaluronidase with local anesthesia in ophthalmology: preliminary report. *Arch Ophthalmol.* 1949; 42:628–633.

58   Hustead, Robert F. Personal communication.

59   Kallio H, Paloheimo M, Maunuksela E-L. Hyaluronidase as an adjuvant in bupivacaine-lidocaine mixture for retrobulbar/peribulbar block. *Anesth Analg.* 2000; 91:934–937.

60   Fanning GL. Hyaluronidase in ophthalmic anesthesia (letter). *Anesth Analg.* 2001; 92:560.

61   Bowman RJ. Is hyaluronidase helpful for peribulbar anaesthesia? *Eye.* 1997; 11:385–388.

62   Dempsey GA. Hyaluronidase and peribulbar block. *Br J Anaesth.* 1997; 78:671–674.

63   Brown SM, Brooks SE, Mazow ML, Avilla CW, Braverman DE, Greenshaw ST, Green ME, McCartney DL, Tabin GC. Cluster of diplopia cases after periocular anesthesia without hyaluronidase. *J Cataract Refract Surg.* 1999; 25:1245–1249.

64   Troll G, Borodic G. Diplopia after cataract surgery using 4% lidocaine in the absence of Wydase (sodium hyaluronidase) [letter]. *J Clin Anesth.* 1999; 11:615–616.

65   Guise P, Laurent S. Sub-tenon's block: The effect of hyaluronidase on speed of onset and block quality. *Anaesth Intensive Care.* 1999; 27:179–181.

66   Rowley SA, Hale JE, Finlay RD. Sub-Tenon's local anaesthesia: the effect of hyaluronidase. *Br J Ophthalmol.* 2000; 84:435–436.

67   Zahl K, Jordan A, Soresen B, Gotta. pH-adjusted lidocaine/bupivacaine mixture are superior for peribulbar block. *Anesthesiology.* 1988; 69:A368.

68   Zahl K, Jordan A, McGroarty J, Gotta A. pH-adjusted bupivacaine and hyaluronidase for peribulbar block. *Anesthesiology.* 1990; 72:230–232.

69   Moharib MM, Anaesth M, Mitra S. Alkalinized lidocaine and bupivacaine with hyaluronidase for sub-Tenon's ophthalmic block. *Reg Anesth Pain Med.* 2000; 25:514–517.

70   Nørregaard JC, Schein OD, Bellan L, Black C, Alonso J, Bernth-Petersen P, Dunn E, Andersen TF, Espallargues M, Anderson GF. International variation in anesthesia care during cataract surgery: results from the International Cataract Surgery Outcomes Study. *Arch Ophthalmol.* 1997; 115:1304–1308.

71   Pecka SL, Dexter F. Anesthesia providers' interventions during cataract extraction under monitored anesthesia care. *AANA J* 1997; 65:357–360.

72   Kumar CM, Lawler PG. Pulmonary oedema after peribulbar block. *Br J Anaesth.* 1999; 82:777–779.

7

Topical Anaesthesia

Dr Gary L. Fanning
Dr Richard A. Fichman

History

The history of topical anaesthesia for ophthalmic surgery begins with the dawning of local anaesthesia itself. In 1884 Koller[1,2] demonstrated the use of topical cocaine for ophthalmic surgery, which opened the age of topical and regional anaesthesia at a time when general anaesthesia was still in its infancy. Soon after this, injection techniques of local anaesthesia became popular, and regional and general anaesthesia remained predominant for eye surgery for a hundred years. Prior to modern surgical techniques for cataract surgery, surgeons needed and demanded absolute akinesia of the eye. Late in the 20th century a return to topical anaesthesia for more complex operations on the eye became possible. Advances in microsurgery for cataract extraction allowed smaller incisions and greater control of the optic media and the intraocular pressure. In 1991 Fichman[3] reported the use of topical anaesthesia for clear-corneal cataract extractions and started a revolution in anaesthesia for cataract surgery.

Anatomy and Pharmacology

The cornea receives its innervation from branches of the ophthalmic division of the trigeminal nerve that reach the globe through the long ciliary nerves. The terminal branches pass among the epithelial cells of the cornea to form the intraepithelial plexus. In this superficial location the nerve cells are naked[4] and are especially vulnerable to the effects of topical anaesthetics. Sensory branches of the trigeminal nerve also reach the iris and sclera by way of the long ciliary nerves. Innervation of the conjunctiva is more complex, as numerous branches of the ophthalmic division of the trigeminal nerve contribute to it. Nonetheless, the nerve endings are quite superficial and local anaesthetics are easily absorbed through this mucous membrane.

Absorption of local anaesthetics through the corneal epithelium and conjunctiva is rapid and effective. A variety of local anaesthetics can be used to produce excellent topical anaesthesia, although some appear to be more desirable than others. Due to their rapid absorption and onset of action, ester-linked anaesthetics, such as tetracaine and proparacaine, have enjoyed a prominent role in topical anaesthesia for the eye[5] for a long time. The amide-linked agents, lidocaine and bupivacaine, have increased in popularity more recently in conjunction with topical anaesthesia for cataract surgery. These agents are absorbed more slowly, but their durations of action are more prolonged.[6]

Diffusion of local anaesthetics through tissues is determined by the concentration of the base form of the anaesthetic present.[7] In most tissues, buffering capacity is adequate to ensure that a high enough concentration of base is formed to reach the nerve endings. In mucous membranes, however, there is not enough buffering capacity to ensure this. To improve topical anaesthesia one can either buffer the anaesthetic before applying or apply a higher concentration than used for injection. Thus one normally uses 2–4% lidocaine for topical anaesthesia instead of the 1–1.5% used for injection techniques. Unbuffered procaine is a poor topical anaesthetic, because its pK_a is so high (8.9) that only 3% of the drug is present in base form at pH 7.4 (compared with 29% for lidocaine, whose pK_a is 7.8, and 17% for bupivacaine, whose pK_a is 8.1). Sun et al.[6] noted that buffered solutions of lidocaine and bupivacaine have longer anaesthetic effects than either procaine or benzocaine, noting as well that all four had anaesthetic effects within a minute of instillation.

Advantages of Topical Anaesthesia

Practitioners who for many years strove for ideal conditions for cataract surgery (i.e., complete anaesthesia and akinesia) might wonder why one would wish to use topical anaesthesia for complex ocular surgery at all. In truth, topical anaesthesia offers several advantages over injection techniques. It is quick, non-invasive, and generally well tolerated by patients. It completely avoids many of the rare but serious complications of orbital regional blocks, such as retrobulbar haemorrhage, postoperative strabismus, optic nerve damage, brainstem anaesthesia, and globe perforation. Although some surgeons still prefer an akinetic eye, others appreciate having motility spared, so that they can ask the patient to gaze in specific directions in order to facilitate the surgery. Patients like the 'no-shot' aspect of topical anaesthesia, enjoy the immediate improvement in vision, and delight in not having to wear a patch. With less invasive methods of cataract extraction and intraocular lens implantation continuing to evolve, it is nearly certain that topical anaesthesia will play an even more important role than it already does. According to Leaming,[8] who annually polls the members of the American Society of Cataract and Refractive Surgery, over 40% of the members now primarily use topical anaesthesia for cataract surgery. Whilst many studies have shown that patients have more sensation during topical anaesthesia than with an orbital regional block, the overwhelming conclusion is that more than 95%

of patients would choose to have their second cataract operation performed under topical anaesthesia as well.[9,10]

Patient Selection for Topical Anaesthesia

Not all patients are appropriate candidates for cataract surgery under topical anesthesia.[11] The ideal candidate is highly motivated, unafraid, and insightful. This patient would have no crippling psychological problems, possess excellent communication skills, and have no unusual problems within the eye that might require a more invasive surgical procedure. Thus patients who suffer dementia, mental retardation, hysteria or extreme anxiety, extreme claustrophobia, immaturity (i.e., children), communication difficulties (i.e., deafness, language barriers, post-stroke aphasia), and/or nystagmus are unsuitable candidates for topical anaesthesia. It has been interesting, however, that most surgeons who enjoy doing cataract surgery under topical anaesthesia have found that their criteria for exclusion have dwindled as their experience grows. For example, if the surgeon and surgical team are willing to make the effort, many problems stemming from communication barriers came be overcome. Deaf patients can be taught hand signals, patients with language barriers can provide or be provided with interpreters, and patients with expressive but not receptive aphasia may be perfectly cooperative and may be able to use hand signals. With experience and motivation, the majority of patients who are appropriate candidates for orbital regional anaesthesia are also candidates for topical anaesthesia and there are surgeons who are doing over 90% of their patients with topical anaesthesia.

Some simple tests have been suggested to determine whether or not a patient is going to be a good candidate for topical anaesthesia. Fraser et al.[12] devised a scoring system following tonometry and A-scan analysis of axial length. They were able to determine that the scores achieved during tonometry and the A-scan correlated very well with the patient's behaviour during surgery. Dinsmore[13] uses a 'drop, then decide' approach, in which surgery is begun under topical with mild intravenous sedation. The patient's response early in the case determines whether or not to proceed under topical. They were successful (i.e., not having to do an orbital regional anaesthetic) in cataract surgery 92% of the time using this strategy.

Communication

An information barrage should begin as soon as surgery is scheduled. Knowing what to expect and having realistic expectations are key to the patient (and thus the surgeon) having a positive experience. In addition to the surgeon's initial description of the procedure, the patient should receive adequate audiovisual and printed information to answer all questions. It is useful for patients to be told that with topical anaesthesia they become important members of the team and that they will be helping the surgeon by being able to move the eye as required during the surgery. On the day of surgery, the surgical team must reinforce all this information, telling patients that the surgeon will ask them to look up or down, right or left, or to stare straight ahead at the light on the microscope (which should be sufficiently dimmed to improve patient comfort without compromising the surgeon's view). Patients must also understand that they may feel pressure or vibration during the surgery as well as the movement of the surgeon's hands. Reassuring them that the fluid they may feel dripping is irrigation fluid and not their own blood is also very helpful. As they often anticipate that they must hold their eyelids open, patients should be informed about the lid speculum and about the permissibility of blinking during surgery. Patients need to know that any discomfort experienced should be communicated to the team at once, either by speaking up or by squeezing someone's hand. It is comforting for patients to understand that pain is not expected and that there is something which can be done should it occur. Many patients are afraid of sneezing or coughing during the operation. Relief of this fear is easily achieved by providing a caregiver to hold the patient's hand. Squeezing the hand is a signal that something is amiss — pain, a cough or a sneeze coming on, a cramp in a calf muscle, etc. — and that surgery should be temporarily halted. Although patients can be coached to speak up if such events occur, having a hand to hold is an extraordinarily comforting feeling, one that is worth more than gallons of potent sedatives.

Communication by the surgeon during the procedure is of particular benefit to patients having surgery under topical anaesthesia. Focusing on the surgeon's voice and hearing what is transpiring can turn the patient's attention away from minor discomforts that would otherwise be a problem. It adds to the patients' feelings of security to hear their surgeon speaking directly to them and leaves them feeling that they were treated as a person and not an object. All conversation in the room should be patient-centred or at least involve the patient as one of the participants in the discussion. Whilst this is important advice for treating patients who are wide awake during surgery, it is especially sound advice for the topical patient. One must never underestimate the importance of good communication and the potential harm of poor.

Patient Preparation

As in all surgeries it is wise to begin by looking at the patient's history and physical examination, checking especially for current medications, compliance and allergies. Always examine the eye to be certain that no acute infectious processes are present that might require cancellation of the procedure. Once the vital signs have been taken and recorded, it is appropriate to begin mydriatic eye drops. Opinions differ regarding the patient with a non-dilating pupil. Some feel that a small pupil is a relatively strong contraindication to topical anaesthesia, whilst others are quite comfortable using physical means to dilate the pupil under topical.[9] If the surgeon is of the former opinion, it is necessary to see if the pupil will adequately dilate (usually 5 mm or more) before proceeding under topical.

A variety of anaesthetic eye drops have been used for topical anaesthesia for cataract surgery, including 0.5% tetracaine, 0.5% proparacaine, 4% lidocaine, and

0.75% bupivacaine. Of these drops proparacaine seems to produce the least amount of stinging on application[14] and can be used alone or to precede others. Other strategies to reduce stinging include using diluted drops initially[15] (one tenth or less of their working strength) and/or warming the drops to about 35° C. In some institutions the topical is applied in the operating theatre right before prepping and draping. In others the drops are begun in a holding area or preparation room and continued periodically prior to the operating theatre. This is helpful if lidocaine or bupivacaine are used, as they often take longer to have their full effect. Both of these have longer durations of action than either proparacaine or tetracaine but still much shorter than their durations when given by injection. As all of these agents work well, the ultimate choice should be made by the surgeon and/or anaesthetist.

Sedation

For many surgeons sedation is an important part of the topical technique, whilst for others it plays a minor role or is avoided altogether. Before completely dismissing the use of sedation, however, one must consider that a large proportion of patients having cataract surgery are significantly anxious. During a recent quality assessment exercise at the Hauser-Ross Eye Institute (unpublished data), it was discovered that patients having topical anaesthesia were significantly more anxious in the operating room than were patients having orbital regional blocks. In the subjective part of the study the patients self-scored using a visual analogue scale. There was objective confirmation from the significantly greater need for both sedation and for blood pressure control in the topical patients compared with the block patients.

As discussed above, communication is an important part of topical anaesthesia. Replacing communication with sedation can be counterproductive and even harmful if a patient reacts inappropriately or suffers a side effect (apnoea, nausea, restlessness, etc.) as a result of using sedation during the surgical procedure. On the other hand, some surgeons like to incorporate substantial amounts of rapid, short-acting sedatives into their technique whilst using minimal amounts of topical anaesthesia.[16] The authors favour using small amounts of sedation for those patients who display significant anxiety. The goal is to make the patient feel comfortable and relaxed. At times it might be necessary to assist a patient having noticeable discomfort by giving small amounts of agents such as propofol, thiopentone, midazolam, or opioids. However, every effort should be taken to prevent over sedation and to rely as much as possible on small doses combined with good communication and reassurance. As will be noted below, the use of intracameral lidocaine may also be used to reduce intraoperative discomfort without having to resort to sedation.

Variations of Topical Anaesthesia

Whilst many surgeons have been satisfied with simply using topical anaesthetic drops with or without sedation, others have devised a variety of adjunctive methods to increase their satisfaction and that of their patients. The following will outline but a few of these methods.

Bloomberg Ophthalmic Ring

Dr Leroy Bloomberg[17] developed and patented a spongiform ring that is intended to be saturated in anaesthetic solution and placed on the eye during surgery. The ring is of sufficient diameter that the corneal limbus is free for the surgical approach. By keeping the ring saturated with anaesthetic during the surgery topical anaesthesia can be maintained for very long periods without dropping anaesthetic directly on the cornea.

Rosenthal Deep Topical, Fornix Applied, Pressurized, Anaesthesia

Dr Kenneth Rosenthal[18] uses a technique that he calls deep topical, fornix applied, pressurized, nerve-block anaesthesia. In this method of topical, two small sponges are soaked in anaesthetic and tucked into the superior and inferior fornices, after which a Honan balloon is placed over the closed eye and pressurized to 30–35 mm Hg for 10–15 minutes. The sponges are removed prior to the onset of surgery. The rationale for this technique lies in anaesthetising the nerves to the cornea and conjunctiva more posteriorly using external pressure to increase the tissue pressure gradient favouring movement of the anaesthetic molecules deep into the tissues. Using this method, Rosenthal finds that the degree of anaesthesia mimics that of a retrobulbar block, hence his use of the term 'nerve-block anaesthesia.'

Following the initial experience with the Rosenthal technique when doing topical anaesthesia at the Hauser-Ross Eye Institute, several complications occurred. A number of corneal abrasions occurred, most of which were felt to be due to the patient's moving the eye around under the Honan balloon, thereby displacing the sponge and scraping the cornea. In a few instances, removal of the sponges at the time of surgery was difficult in patients with very deep fornices. Finally, the only adult patient exhibiting a classic oculocardiac reflex in ten years at our institution was one in whom the Honan balloon was inflated after placement of the sponges in the fornices. In spite of these problems, it remains a very useful and popular method for obtaining excellent topical anaesthesia.

Topical Anaesthesia Combined with Perilimbal Anaesthesia

A number of surgeons have used a combined approach, following topical anaesthesia with a low-volume (often 1 ml or less) perilimbal subconjunctival injection of local anaesthetic, such as described by Pallan et al.[19] Many surgeons use this technique to perform pain-free scleral tunnel incisions. For clear-corneal incisions supplementation with a perilimbal injection is seldom necessary.

Intracameral Local Anaesthetics

Since Dr Richard Fitchman[20] first noted that a small amount of preservative-free tetracaine injected into the anterior chamber eliminated pain associated with iris chafing, intracameral injection of local anaesthetic has become one of the most widely used adjuncts to topical anaesthesia for cataract surgery. Gills et al.[21,22] observed that some patients complained of pressure or pain during cataract surgery under topical anaesthesia. He studied two groups of patients, one in which he injected balanced salt solution (BSS) intracamerally and another in which he used 1% preservative-free lidocaine. When using 0.5 ml of 1% lidocaine, the incidence of discomfort was reduced to 3% compared with an incidence of 26% in his control group (BSS). They reported no ill effects from 1% lidocaine used in this fashion. Others have confirmed the efficacy of this method in reducing discomfort during anterior segment surgery under topical anaesthesia.[23–26]

Is it Safe to Inject Local Anaesthetic into the Anterior Chamber?
A number of groups have attempted to answer this question, both in human and experimental models. Kim et al.[27] in an in vitro study of rabbit and human corneas found that both BSS and 1% lidocaine produce transient oedema of the corneal endothelium, which readily reversed when the perfusion was ended. Eggeling et al.[28] studied the effects of BSS and preservative-free lidocaine in concentrations of 1%, 5%, and 10% on porcine corneas over time. After up to 60 minutes of perfusion, 1% lidocaine caused no more damage than BSS. The higher concentrations, however, caused significant endothelial cell loss. Kadonosono et al.[29] looked at the effects of three concentrations of preservative-free lidocaine, 0.02%, 0.2%, and 2%, on the corneal endothelium of rabbits. In each animal the fellow eye was injected with BSS as a control. They found that 2% lidocaine altered the shapes of these endothelial cells and resulted in the loss of microvilli. They concluded that the low concentrations used clinically were safe but that higher concentrations risked damaging the corneal epithelium. Finally, Anderson et al.[30] compared the effects of bupivacaine and lidocaine injected intracamerally in patients and did a laboratory study using rabbit corneas. Comparing 0.5% bupivacaine and 1% lidocaine in patients, both were found to be equally safe and effective. In the rabbit model, however, bupivacaine caused significant endothelial cell damage, which could be prevented by diluting the bupivacaine 1:1 with glutathione bicarbonate Ringer solution. In summary, to date virtually all studies have shown that preservative-free 1% lidocaine is safe when injected in small volumes (0.5 ml) into the anterior chamber.

What Happens if there is a Tear in the Posterior Capsule and Lidocaine Solution Diffuses into the Vitreous?
Gills et al.[22] reported amaurosis in four patients following the use of intracameral lidocaine and that in each case the posterior capsule was not intact. All four patients recovered completely within hours. Gills rightfully points out, however, that one should not automatically ascribe postoperative amaurosis following surgery under topical anaesthesia to the migration of lidocaine into the vitreous. As this is a very rare event, other more serious causes of amaurosis, such as retinovascular or cerebrovascular occlusion or other occurrences must be investigated.

Lidocaine Gel

The search continues for an ideal topical anaesthetic. Several groups have started using 2% lidocaine gel as their agent of choice. Barequet et al.[31] at the Wilmer Eye Institute in Baltimore compared this agent with 0.5% tetracaine drops and found that both achieved similar results in patients. Studies on rabbit corneas indicated no clinically evident nor histopathologically discernable tissue damage resulting from the lidocaine gel, including three rabbits in which intentional intracameral injection of the gel was carried out. Assia et al.[32] also reported using lidocaine gel and found it to be both safe and effective in a group of 100 patients. Harman[33] found the use of lidocaine gel to be equally effective as tetracaine. In clinical use the gel is applied into the fornices and the eyelid taped shut until the patient is ready for surgery. Rinsing of the residual gel is not a problem, and Assia and co-workers reported that the gel provided prolonged lubrication and facilitated the surgery.

Conclusions

Whilst the specific technical aspects of performing surgery under topical anaesthesia have not been mentioned in this chapter, they have been well covered in previous publications.[11,34,35] There is a definite learning curve associated with this technique, both for the surgeon and for the surgical team. Adhering to rather rigid guidelines for selecting and managing patients, especially insisting upon good communication, will help ensure success. Initially it will seem strange to be operating on a patient whose eye is free to move and who is able to see immediately after surgery. Before very long, however, it will seem natural and desirable for everyone involved. Complications may occur which will necessitate switching to orbital regional anaesthesia, but these cases will be rare with experience and proper patient selection.

Topical anaesthesia for anterior segment surgery is now an extremely important modality, one that continues to grow in popularity. There is little doubt about its importance in the future as improvements in surgical technique, in topical anaesthetic agents, and in the availability of more specific anxiolytic agents take place. Whilst this form of anaesthesia may not be desirable for all surgeons and all patients at present, the proportion of patients undergoing cataract surgery using other forms of anaesthesia will continue to fall. Knowing the rare but devastating complications of more invasive forms of anaesthesia, it is appropriate that topical anaesthesia becomes predominant in uncomplicated cataract surgery.

References

1   Knapp H. On cocaine and its use in ophthalmic and general surgery. *Arch Ophthalmol.* 1884; 13:402.
2   Koller K. Preliminary report on local anesthesia of the eye: Translation of classic paper originally published in 1884. *Arch Ophthalmol.* 1934; 12:473–474.
3   Fichman RA. Topical eye drops replace injection for anesthesia. *Ocul Surg News.* 1992; 10:1.

4   Snell RS, Lemp MA. *Clinical Anatomy of the Eye*. Blackwell Scientific Publications, Boston, 1989; 132.

5   deJong RH. *Local Anesthetics*. Mosby, St. Louis, 1994. pp 153–154.

6   Sun R, Hamilton RC, Gimbel HV. Comparison of 4 topical anesthetic agents for effect and corneal toxicity in rabbits. *J Cataract Refract Surg.* 1999; 25:1232–1236.

7   deJong RH. *Local Anesthetics*. Mosby, St. Louis, 1994. pp 106–116.

8   Leaming DV. Practice styles and preferences of ASCRS members — 1999 survey. *J Cataract Refract Surg.* 2000; 26:913–921.

9   Mönestam E, Kuusik M, Wachtmeister L. Topical anesthesia for cataract surgery: a population-based perspective. *J Cataract Refract Surg.* 2001; 27:445–451.

10   Zehetmayer M, Radax U, Skorpik C, Menapace R, Schemper M, Weghaupt H, Scholz U. Topical versus peribulbar anesthesia in clear corneal cataract surgery. *J Cataract Refract Surg.* 1996; 22:480–4840.

11   Fichman RA. Topical anesthesia. In: Davis DB, Mandel MR, editors. *Ophthalmology Clinics of North America,* vol. 11. 1998. pp 125–126.

12   Fraser SG, Siriwadena D, Jamieson H, Girault J, Bryan SJ. Indicators of patient suitability for topical anesthesia. *J Cataract Refract Surg.* 1997; 23:781–783.

13   Dinsmore SC. Drop, then decide approach to topical anesthesia. *J Cataract Refract Surg.* 1995; 21:666–671.

14   Hamilton R, Claoue C. Topical anesthesia: Proxymetacaine (proparacaine) versus Amethocaine (tetracaine) for clear corneal phacoemulsification. *J Cataract Refract Surg.* 1998; 24:1382–1384.

15   Hustead RF, Hamilton RC. Pharmacology. In: Gills JP, Hustead RF, Sanders, DR, editors. *Ophthalmic Anesthesia*. Slack Incorporated, Thorofare, NJ, 1993. pp 67–102.

16   Rand WJ, Stein SC, Velazquez GE. Rand–Stein analgesia protocol for cataract surgery. *Ophthalmology.* 2000; 107:889–895.

17   Bloomberg LB, Pellican KJ. Topical anesthesia using the Bloomberg SuperNumb Anesthetic Ring. *J Cataract Refract Surg.* 1995; 21:16–20.

18   Rosenthal KJ. Deep topical, nerve-block anesthesia. *J Cataract Refract Surg.* 1995; 21:499–503.

19   Pallan LA, Kondrot EC, Stout RR. Sutureless scleral tunnel cataract surgery using topical and low dose perilimbal anesthesia. *J Cataract Refract Surg.* 1995; 21:504–507.

20   Fichman RA. Phacoemulsification with topical anesthesia. In: Fine IH, Fichman RA, Grabow HB, editors. *Clear-corneal Cataract Surgery and Topical Anesthesia*. Slack Incorporated, Thorofare, NJ, 1993. p 116.

21   Gills JP, Cherchio M, Raanan MG. Unpreserved lidocaine to control discomfort during cataract surgery using topical anesthesia. *J Cataract Refract Surg.* 1997; 23:545–550.

22   Gills JP, Johnson DE, Cherchio M, Raanan MG. Intraocular anesthesia. In: Davis DB, Mandel MR, editors. *Ophthalmology Clinics of North America,* vol. 11. 1998. pp 65–71.

23   Masket S, Gokmen F. Efficacy and safety of intracameral lidocaine as a supplement to topical anesthesia. *J Cataract Refract Surg.* 1998; 24:956–960.

24   Tseng SH, Chen FK. A randomized clinical trial of combined topical-intracameral anesthesia in cataract surgery. *Ophthalmology.* 1998; 105:2007–2017.

25   Martin RG, Miller JD, Cox CC 3rd Ferrel SC, Raanan MG. Safety and efficacy of intracameral injections of unpreserved lidocaine to reduce intraocular sensation. *J Cataract Refract Surg.* 1998; 24:961–963.

26   Crandall AS, Zabriskie NA, Patel BC, Burns TA, Mamalis N, Malmquist-Carter LA, Yee R. A comparison of patient comfort during cataract surgery with topical anesthesia versus topical anesthesia and intracameral lidocaine. *Ophthalmology.* 1999; 106:60–660.

27   Kim T, Holley GP, Lee JH, Broocker G, Edelhauser HF. The effects of intraocular lidocaine on the corneal endothelium. *Ophthalmology.* 1998; 105:125–130.

28   Eggeling P, Pleyer U, Hartmann C, Rieck PW. Corneal endothelial toxicity of different lidocaine concentrations. *J Cataract Refractive Surg.* 2000; 26:1403–1408.
29   Kadonosono K, Ito N, Yazama F, Nishide T, Sugita M, Sawada H, Ohno S. Effect of intracameral anesthesia on the corneal epithelium. *J Cataract Refract Surg.* 1998; 24:1377–1381.
30   Anderson NJ, Nath R, Anderson CJ, Edelhauser HF. Comparison of preservative-free bupivacaine versus lidocaine for intracameral anesthesia: a randomized clinical trial and in vitro analysis. *Am J Ophthalmol.* 199; 127:393–402.
31   Barequet IS, Soriano ES, Green WR, O'Brien TP. Provision of anesthesia with single application of lidocaine 2% gel. *J Cataract Refract Surg.* 1999; 25:626–631.
32   Assia EI, Pras E, Yehezkel M, Rotenstreich Y, Jager-Roshu S. Topical anesthesia using lidocaine gel for cataract surgery. *J Cataract Refract Surg.* 1999; 25:635–639.
33   Harman DM. Combined sedation and topical anesthesia for cataract surgery. *J Cataract Refract Surg.* 2000; 26:109–113.
34   Fine IH, Fichman RA, Grabow HB, editors. *Clear-corneal Cataract Surgery and Topical anesthesia.* Slack Incorporated, Thorofare, NJ, 1993.
35   Fichman RA. Advances in cataract surgery. *Adv Clin Ophthalmol.* 1995; 2:133–166.

8

Monitored Sedation for Ophthalmic Surgery

Dr Gary L. Fanning

Introduction

The majority of ophthalmic surgery is performed on an outpatient basis, often under local anaesthesia. Providing safe and effective sedation is a very important skill because patients may be apprehensive about having eye surgery and some procedures may be painful. The purpose of this chapter is to review the pharmacology of the agents currently being used for sedation in adults in the outpatient setting and to discuss their uses during ophthalmic surgery. The rapid-acting, short-duration drugs will be emphasized.

Goals of Sedation

In producing sedation, the anaesthetist generally endeavours to achieve anxiolysis, amnesia, and/or somnolence. Providing significant analgesia is an additional goal in many instances. One does not necessarily need to accomplish all of these goals in every patient, although in some instances sedation may be required to a point just short of general anaesthesia, if only briefly. The choice of sedative technique depends on a variety of factors: the patient, the procedure, the surgeon, and safety.

Each patient presents with many variables that will influence these choices. These include age, gender, systemic illnesses, presence or absence of pain, psychopathology, drug use or abuse, allergy, and anaesthetic history. Patients undergoing ophthalmic surgery are likely to be elderly and suffer from multiple systemic illnesses. Failure to consider these variables may result in unpleasant surprises for the anaesthetist and perhaps worse for the patient.[1]

Surgical procedures differ in length, complexity, and degree of discomfort. Short procedures, including routine cataract extraction, may require little or no sedation.

Others, especially those associated with oculoplastic surgery, require rather deep sedation for administration of the local anaesthetic, after which the patient may need to be awake in order to cooperate during the surgery. Patients undergoing longer procedures may benefit by continuous sedation techniques in order to tolerate lying quietly for an extended period of time. The nature of the procedure also dictates the type and degree of sedation required; for example, total lack of movement by the patient may be so essential that only general anaesthesia will assure proper conditions.

The surgeon's preference is an important consideration in the choice of sedation. Some surgeons enjoy talking with their patients during surgery, whilst others demand absolute silence and total lack of movement. It is always important for the whole team to be aware of and respect the surgeon's preferences and, when necessary, to discuss them with the patient. On occasion it is advisable to recommend general anaesthesia for the marginally cooperative patient who is scheduled with a surgeon who poorly tolerates any distraction. In specific cases consultation with the surgeon is helpful.

As in all forms of anaesthesia, patient safety comes first. Sedation must be achieved whilst providing cardio-respiratory stability, good operating conditions, and a rapid return of the patient's preoperative mental and physical activities. Rapid return to full recovery is especially important for the outpatient, who typically goes home without the benefit of the trained observers and specialised facilities available to the hospitalised patient.

Monitoring During Sedation

The American Society of Anaesthesiologists (ASA) first approved standards for basic anaesthesia monitoring in 1986 and amended those standards in 1998.[2] Monitoring begins with the presence of a trained observer in the operating room during the entire procedure. This should apply to all anaesthetic techniques. The anaesthetist responsible for administration of the sedation should be the one monitoring the patient. Surgeons should not perform surgery whilst attempting to direct the administration of sedative agents by personnel who have not been adequately trained in their use.

Oxygenation, ventilation, and circulation should be monitored in patients undergoing surgery. Oximetry and supplemental oxygenation are extremely important, because even healthy individuals can desaturate rapidly after even modest doses of sedatives. Many young and healthy patients may safely breathe room air. Patients with cardio-respiratory disease are prone to desaturate after very small doses of sedatives, including non-opiates.[3] If oxygen must be discontinued (because of the fire hazard), such as during use of electrocautery in oculoplastic surgery, pulse oximetry becomes even more important. Extensive use of cautery requires that the surgical field be prepared in such a way as to prevent the accumulation of oxygen under the drapes.[4]

Ventilation can be monitored by direct observation of the patient's breathing pattern, by a precordial stethoscope, and by capnography. Divided nasal cannulae are available that allow administration of oxygen via one nostril whilst withdrawing air from the other for analysis of expired carbon dioxide. Use of continuous capnography is especially encouraged when continuous sedation techniques are used for longer procedures, such as oculoplastic and retinal operations.

In addition to pulse oximetry, circulation can be monitored by an electrocardiograph, a precordial stethoscope, and a non-invasive blood pressure device. Significant rises or falls in systemic blood pressure may be seen during procedures under local anaesthesia and sedation. Treatment may be necessary, for example, during vitreoretinal (VR) procedures.

Bispectral analysis monitoring is becoming more common. Although it is more often used during general anaesthesia, it has been used as a monitor in the awake patient[5,6] and has been found to be an excellent predictor of the level of sedation.

Basic Pharmacokinetics, Pharmacodynamics, and Synergism

Pharmacokinetics

Ideally one would like to use drugs for sedation in ophthalmic surgery which are rapidly redistributed and eliminated.[7] Not all drugs exhibit both properties, even though they may be quite suitable for outpatient use. For example, midazolam has a redistribution half-life of about 11 minutes, whilst its elimination half-life is about 2 hours. Remifentanil, an extremely rapid and short-acting opioid, has a redistribution half-life of only one minute and an elimination half-life of only nine minutes.

The concept of context-sensitive half-time[8–11] has emerged to describe the pharmacokinetics of many drugs used in anaesthesia. It is the time needed for the plasma concentration of a drug to fall to 50% of a concentration that has been held constant for a specific period of time (the context). For most drugs that we use the context-sensitive half-time increases as duration of administration increases. In some it increases and then plateaus, and in others it remains constant in spite of very long periods of administration (see Figure 1). Knowing the context-sensitive half-time helps predict how quickly a patient will recover following the infusion of a sedative.

Pharmacokinetic parameters vary due to patient and drug characteristics. Age, gender, presence of disease, obesity, and drug history[12] are all important patient factors affecting the body's handling of drugs, whilst the drug factors influencing pharmacokinetics include fat solubility, protein and tissue binding, and susceptibility to enzymatic breakdown.

Pharmacodynamics

Whilst some drugs have an all-or-nothing effect, most of our sedative drugs will exhibit different effects depending on the dose given. For example, thiopentone is a very useful sedative, producing short-lasting effects when given in small doses. Larger doses result in the induction of anaesthesia, whilst still larger doses may result in coma and death. Likewise the opioids may provide analgesia in smaller doses whilst producing profound analgesia, apnoea, and loss of consciousness in higher

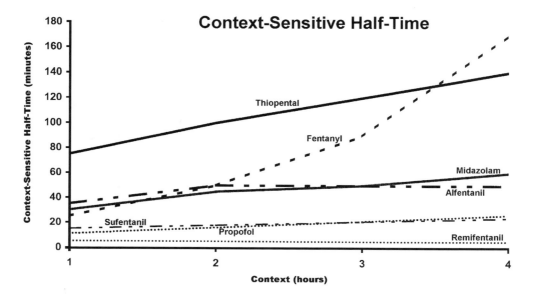

Fig. 1.   Context-sensitive half-time. This chart represents a compilation of figures from a variety of references.[8–11] The values have been rounded for ease of comparison and remembering.

doses. In order to provide safe sedation for our patients, it is essential for us to be aware of differential pharmacodynamics and to adjust doses accordingly.

The effects of many drugs on the body result from the interaction of a drug with a receptor. One of the best known examples is the opioid receptor family. Others include the gamma-aminobutyric acid (GABA) receptors, N-methyl-D-aspartate (NMDA) receptor, and α2-adrenoceptors. Barbiturates, benzodiazepines, etomidate, and propofol interact with the GABA receptor complexes, whilst ketamine and nitrous oxide interact with the NMDA receptor.[13]

Synergism describes the concept that drugs in combination often have greater effects than the sum of the individual doses of the drugs given alone.[14] Whilst this is useful and allows us to reduce the total amount of drug used, complications can also occur more often as the result of synergism. Apnoea and hypoxemia occur twice as often when using the combination of midazolam and fentanyl than when either drug is given alone.[15] Recently Mertens et al.[16] demonstrated that the haemodynamic effects of propofol may alter the pharmacokinetics of simultaneously administered alfentanil so that initial plasma concentrations of alfentanil may be quite higher than expected. It is necessary, therefore, to use great care when administering multiple agents, especially to our elderly patients with multiple systemic illnesses.[17,18]

Methods of Administration

A variety of methods is available to us for administration of sedatives. Sedative goals, duration of surgery, and type of patient all influence which mode of administration will be most useful. In children, for example, oral, nasal, and rectal routes of administering sedatives are quite common. Transmucosal and transdermal routes are also being used.[19,20]

All routes of administration have their advantages and disadvantages. The biggest advantage of the less-invasive routes is that they are less painful than intramuscular or intravenous administration. The biggest disadvantages are lack of reliability and unpredictability. If given too early, the effect can be wearing off by the time the patient needs it. If given too late, the patient may not experience significant sedation until discharged. Nonetheless, oral premedication is quite appropriate in many settings and is used in a variety of ophthalmic surgical situations, including refractive surgery, oculoplastic surgery, and even cataract surgery. The intramuscular route of administration should not be used in the elderly. It is painful and very unpredictable.

The intravenous technique is the most practical method of providing safe, effective, and predictable sedation. With modern agents small doses can be titrated to effect quite reliably. Intermittent boluses are suitable for short procedures, supplemented by fractional doses as needed. In longer cases, continuous infusion techniques are more useful. There are several infusion pumps available that allow very precise dosing based on the patient's body weight. A newer technique for sedation using target-controlled infusion (TCI),[21,22] employs a programmed pump to infuse drugs to a predetermined effect site concentration.[23] Another intravenous method is that of patient-controlled sedation, which has been described for use in patients undergoing peribulbar block.[24–26] The use of either of these techniques combined with bispectral-analysis monitoring may become quite common in the future, especially for longer procedures.

Sedative Agents

Barbiturates

Anaesthetists have used short-acting barbiturates for at least 60 years. Their record of safety and effectiveness is well known. Drugs such as methohexitone and thiopentone are given commonly for a variety of ophthalmic procedures, both to sedate the patient prior to regional anaesthesia and to provide mild sedation and anxiolysis during the surgery itself. Sub-hypnotic doses of these drugs (5–30 mg of methohexitone or 12.5–50 mg of thiopentone) produce a pleasant state of reverie in many patients whilst allowing them to remain cooperative and quiet. Slightly higher doses may be needed in large, younger patients or patients who are excessively anxious. Their onset of action is very fast, and in small doses the effects are short lasting. Circulatory and respiratory stability are maintained with these doses, unlike the effects of the higher doses used to induce general anaesthesia.

Serious untoward effects are rare with the use of sedative doses of barbiturates, but some side effects can be bothersome. Whilst uncommon, some patients complain of severe nausea and vomiting. Sneezing, coughing, hiccoughing, and laryngospasm can also occur, but these phenomena are generally short lasting. Continued administration of a barbiturate should be avoided if such a side effect has occurred. Barbiturates may be antanalgesic and increase the withdrawal response to noxious stimuli. Hence some practitioners combine a smaller dose of barbiturate with a small dose of opioid in order to minimise these unwanted effects, but this often produces respiratory depression.

In a high-volume practice a significant advantage of the short-acting barbiturates is their low cost compared with other agents.

Benzodiazepines

Parenteral benzodiazepines are valuable agents whose effects include amnesia, anxiolysis, muscle relaxation, and somnolence. They are potent anticonvulsants and are particularly useful for treating seizures due to local anaesthetic toxicity. The sedative effects of benzodiazepines result from their agonistic interaction with specific receptor sites on the GABA[1] receptor complex in the central nervous system.[13]

The respiratory effects of benzodiazepines are dose and patient dependent. In healthy, young adults, small doses have no clinically significant respiratory effects, whilst larger doses blunt the hypoxic respiratory drive. Elderly patients, however, are less tolerant and will exhibit respiratory depression at much smaller doses.[27] Patients with sleep apnoea or chronic obstructive pulmonary disease are also more susceptible to the respiratory depressant effects, especially those who exhibit an hypoxic drive.[12] In many patients, as the result of synergism, respiratory depression much greater than expected will occur when these drugs are mixed with opioids, barbiturates, or propofol.

Somnolence, anxiolysis, and amnesia can be reliably produced by benzodiazepines but not to equal degrees by all of the agents in this class. Anxiolysis and amnesia are generally produced at lower doses than significant somnolence. Midazolam, for example, produces amnesia at one tenth the dose required to produce sedation.[9] The amnesic effects vary from patient to patient, but all patients should be given postoperative instructions in writing as well as orally, preferably with a family member or carer present.[28] Whilst some have ascribed postoperative cognitive dysfunction in part due to the use of benzodiazepines,[29] others have been unable to show this.[30,31]

Diazepam has been long used as a premedication and is still used frequently to calm patients prior to refractive surgery procedures. It is predictably absorbed from the GI tract, peaking in about one hour after ingestion but the dose required is unpredictable. Elderly patients may be sedated with as little as 2 mg orally, whilst anxious young adults may require 20 mg or more to achieve the same effect. It should not be administered by the IM route. It is quite painful when injected intravenously and should be preceded by a small dose of lidocaine and be injected into a large vein with freely flowing IV fluid. Even using these precautions, phlebitis may occur.

Because its onset of action is not rapid and its elimination half-life (20–40 hours) is very long, diazepam is not an ideal drug to be used this way in outpatients. One of the products of the degradation of diazepam is oxazepam, a commercially available potent sedative-hypnotic. For these reasons, the use of intravenous diazepam has declined.

Midazolam's pharmacokinetic profile is better than that of diazepam, making it a more desirable drug for outpatient use.[32] It is currently the benzodiazepine of choice in that setting. Its elimination half-life is only about two hours, and its hepatic clearance is virtually 10 times faster than that of diazepam. Its principal metabolite is only one-tenth as potent as the parent compound. It is water-soluble and when given intravenously has a low incidence of sequellae.

Midazolam works rapidly intravenously and has better amnesic properties than diazepam. The peak effect of a small intravenous dose usually occurs within 1–2 minutes. It is wise to wait and measure that effect before giving additional doses or adding significant doses of adjuncts, such as barbiturates, opioids, or propofol. Doses of 0.5–1.0 mg should be the initial amount given to the elderly patient. This dose can be repeated or additional agents may be given as necessary. It can be used in longer cases as a constant infusion of 0.2–3.0 μg/kg/minute. Rapid infusion of large doses of this drug has resulted in respiratory arrest,[28] but this should be a very rare event if care is given during its administration and if vigilance is maintained for synergism when adjuncts are given simultaneously.

Opioid Analgesics
Virtually all of the clinically-important effects of opioids result from the interaction of these drugs with the endogenous μ-receptors in the brain and spinal cord.[32] Analgesia is dose-dependent but does occur at doses which do not produce clinically significant respiratory depression. There is no pure opioid agonist that has significantly fewer side effects than any other when given in equi-analgesic doses. Mixed agonist-antagonist drugs are less likely to produce respiratory depression, but their analgesic effects tend to plateau and their pharmacokinetic profiles make them hard to use. Opioid analgesics are potent respiratory depressants, especially if they have been combined with other agents. Proper attention, monitoring, and the administration of supplemental oxygen are all essential when using these drugs.

Modest doses of intravenous opioids in supine patients seldom produce significant cardiovascular depression. Vagally mediated bradycardia can be seen, but this is easily overcome with glycopyrrolate. Especially apprehensive patients who present with elevated blood pressures often have their pressures reduced to more acceptable levels with a small dose of opioid. In spite of the cardiovascular stability of these drugs, cardiovascular collapse can occur if severe respiratory depression goes untreated.

Opioids are well known for their ability to induce nausea and/or vomiting. This effect is enhanced by vestibular stimulation.[33] Thus, whilst nausea and vomiting are quite uncommon in the supine patient lying quietly, they occur at rates as high as 40% and 15%, respectively, in the ambulatory patient.[34] It is useful, therefore, to use opioids that wear off quickly and to allow patients to recover before being moved from the supine position. Prevention/treatment of opioid-induced nausea and vomiting is usually successful using a butyrophenone, such as droperidol, and/or a serotonin antagonist, such as ondansetron. Droperidol remains the less expensive of the two but has a greater potential for causing side effects and delayed discharge.[35]

A serious side effect associated with the use of rapidly acting opioids is skeletal muscle rigidity[33]. This rare phenomenon is troublesome because the rigidity may make it impossible to ventilate the patient. It is seen most commonly when large intravenous doses are given rapidly, but one must be aware of it and look for it even when giving small doses. It can be overcome by the intravenous administration of an opioid antagonist or by giving succinylcholine. Opioids should only be administered by trained personnel who are familiar with their effects. Some of the longer-acting opioids, such as morphine and pethidine (meperidine), can cause histamine release. The newer opioids, discussed below, have not been associated with this side effect.[33]

Fentanyl was the first of the modern opioids. It has a rapid onset of action and short duration, and its potency is 50–100 times that of morphine. Given in small doses (1–3 µg/kg) its effect is short lasting owing to rapid redistribution. When administered over a prolonged period of time it becomes a longer-acting agent because of its long elimination half-life. In Figure 1 the context-sensitive half-time of fentanyl is seen in contrast with other agents, and its prolongation of duration can be appreciated. It probably should not be used as a continuous infusion in outpatients as there are better drugs available. Fentanyl can produce significant histamine release. The effect of the usual dose (25–50 µg) given to an elderly patient usually peaks in about 3–5 minutes. Fentanyl is easily absorbed through the oral mucosa, and a lollipop (Oralet®) is commercially available that can be used to sedate both children and adults and to treat 'breakthrough' cancer pain.[19,20] The Oralet® has also been used as a premedication for patients undergoing cataract surgery under topical anaesthesia.[36] Unfortunately all of the potential side effects of opioids can still occur even when given in such a seemingly innocuous fashion. The drug is also available in a transdermal preparation for prolonged use.

Sufentanil has a shorter duration of action than fentanyl and is 5–10 times as potent. Boluses of 5–20 µg can be used for sedation in the elderly. It is also useful as a continuous infusion at rates varying from 0.005–0.01 µg/kg/minute. As its context-sensitive half-time is much better than either fentanyl or alfentanil (see Figure 1), it is useful for 2–3 hour cases.

Alfentanil is about 5 times less potent than fentanyl, but it is more rapid in onset and has a shorter duration of action. Taking effect in about 1–2 minutes after bolus injection, it lasts for about 15–20 minutes. In younger patients boluses in the range of 250–500 µg may be appropriate, although only half this much should be given to the elderly or when adjuncts are used. This drug is popular in ophthalmic anaesthesia, and its use alone has compared well with methohexitone for sedation prior to retrobulbar blocks.[37] The author has found it particularly useful in longer cases, such as retinal surgery, where intermittent boluses or a continuous infusion in the order of 0.20–0.30 µg/kg/minute provides conscious sedation. Small doses of midazolam (1–2 mg) at the beginning of the procedure are also given, and respiratory depression has not been a problem in these patients at these doses. Alfentanil may be associated with significantly less nausea and vomiting in the ambulatory patient than either fentanyl or sufentanil.[38]

Remifentanil is very rapidly metabolised by blood and tissue esterases (not the esterases responsible for the metabolism of succinylcholine). As a result, its duration of action is very short and very predictable. About 10–20 times more potent than alfentanil,[39] its onset of action occurs within 1–2 minutes, and its elimination half-time is only 8–10 minutes. Due to its unique mode of elimination, it has a very flat context-sensitive half-time, only 3–4 minutes, which remains constant no matter how long the infusion lasts. Thus 50% reduction of the plasma concentration occurs in 3–4 minutes in cases lasting either one hour or eight hours when the infusion is stopped. Initially remifentanil was not recommended for bolus injection, but in clinical practice this mode of use has been very beneficial. Given in doses of 0.2 μg/kg (slightly higher in young, vigorous patients), a brief period of profound analgesia is produced which gives excellent conditions for the performance of painful blocks as in oculoplastic procedures. It is necessary to thoroughly preoxygenate the patient prior to giving the bolus as the patients frequently develop a short period of apnoea when remifentanil is given. The apnoea is so brief that hypercarbia is not a problem, but significant hypoxaemia can occur if preoxygenation is omitted. Infusions of remifentanil in the range of 0.025–0.1 μg/kg/minute provide excellent continuous sedation in patients needing it for more prolonged procedures. Lower doses are especially important in the elderly and in patients receiving other sedatives. This drug is very potent and can produce apnoea very quickly, making unwavering vigilance absolutely necessary. Whilst expensive, it can be used in a cost-effective manner if it is diluted in such a way that it can be used for more than one patient.

Propofol

Propofol is used to induce and maintain general anaesthesia, to provide long-term sedation in the intensive care unit, and to provide short-term sedation in a variety of settings. Its popularity in the outpatient setting stems from three very important properties: 1) rapid onset, 2) short duration of action, and 3) low incidence of nausea and vomiting. Insoluble in water, it comes prepared in a lipid emulsion containing egg phosphatide, soya bean oil, and glycerol. It is an excellent culture media, so meticulous attention to sterile technique should be followed when preparing and using it. Leftover solution should be discarded after about 6 hours.

Propofol is very rapidly redistributed upon injection and its elimination half-life is very short. It has a huge volume of distribution but an equally large clearance.[32] Whilst its onset of action is not as fast as the short-acting barbiturates, it is still acceptably rapid. Occasionally it takes 45 seconds to see much of a response, so it is wise to be cautious before giving additional doses. Its context-sensitive half-time is longer than remifentanil's, about 10–20 minutes, and it increases only slowly over time. As a result, rapid recovery can be expected even after 3–4 hours of infusion.

Propofol is painful on injection, but there are several strategies to reduce this occurrence: 1) inject into a large vein with freely flowing IV fluid, 2) inject slowly,

3) precede the injection with a small bolus (50 mg) of lidocaine or simply add 10–50 mg of preservative-free lidocaine to a 20-ml vial.[40]

It is a respiratory depressant, particularly to the hypoxic drive,[3] and is notably synergistic with other agents in this capacity. In smaller, sedative doses this is generally not a problem, but the usual monitoring and vigilance are still warranted.

Systolic blood pressure can drop rather significantly with this drug, due both to peripheral vasodilatation and myocardial depression. This effect is common in the elderly, especially with doses that induce general anaesthesia. Dosage control, slow injection, and careful monitoring will minimize this effect. During continuous infusion, the vital signs tend to remain remarkably stable.

Propofol's dose–response curve seems to be wide, making it a little difficult to predict a specific effective dose in a given patient. For example, the induction dose in a child may be 2–3 mg/kg, in a healthy adult 2–2.5 mg/kg, and in the elderly only 0.5–1 mg/kg. The same general rule is true of sedative doses, so that whilst younger adults require 50–100 mg for sedation, the elderly may need 20–30 mg or less. Wide variations in the doses required for continuous sedation also occur and vary from 10–20 µg/kg/minute to 50–75 µg/kg/minute. When using propofol in bolus doses prior to performance of a block, it is frequent to see unwanted movement in younger patients. It is possible to prevent or moderate this by giving a small dose of opioid along with propofol, but one must then watch carefully for respiratory depression.

Propofol reduces intraocular pressure (IOP). Neel et al.[41] showed that a dose of 1.0 mg/kg given to sedate patients prior to orbital blocks resulted in a fall of 17–27% in IOP in the unblocked eye. Likewise, Ferrari and Donlon[42] found lower IOPs after propofol than after methohexitone and midazolam.

One of the hallmarks of propofol is its patient's acceptance. Patients frequently recover from this agent feeling quite well, even euphoric. Nausea is rare, vomiting even rarer. Studies have shown that other agents can achieve equally rapid recovery times, and often more economically,[43] but it is difficult to deny the improved quality of recovery with propofol when compared with others.[44]

Other Agents

Ketamine, a phencyclidine derivative, enjoyed a flurry of popularity when it was introduced 30 years ago, but its use decreased due to the unwanted side effect of hallucinations that was observed in many adult patients during recovery.[9] The drug is making a substantial comeback, especially in outpatient surgery, because it has been found to be a very effective sedative when used in low doses.

In large doses ketamine produces tachycardia and hypertension, effects that can be potentially hazardous to patients with significant coronary artery disease. Fortunately these effects are less pronounced when small, sub-anaesthetic doses are used for sedation. Respiration tends to be very well maintained, as is the airway. Secretions can be a problem, however, and it is helpful to premedicate the patient with an intravenous anticholinergic, such as glycopyrrolate. Nausea and vomiting postoperatively can also be a problem, but prophylactic antiemetic therapy, as mentioned for opioids, is quite effective. Modest increases in intraocular pressure may be seen with ketamine,[45] but this is seldom a problem clinically.

Benzodiazepines, in modest doses, prevent the postoperative hallucinations caused by ketamine. Giving the patient 2 mg of midazolam intravenously and supplementing it with 0.5–1.0 mg periodically during longer procedures nearly assures the absence of hallucinations. Diazepam has been used instead of midazolam,[46] but midazolam has been described more frequently in recent publications.[47,48]

Ketamine in sub-anaesthetic doses is an excellent analgesic, making it a very reasonable choice for sedation prior to painful blocks. Whilst the dose will vary from patient to patient, 10–20 mg increments given to effect will often suffice for very brief, painful procedures when combined with midazolam. Given in this way the patient's airway and cardiovascular stability are both very well maintained. The effects of small doses tend to last 15–20 minutes.

The combination of midazolam–ketamine has been compared with methohexitone for sedating patients prior to peribulbar block. Rosenberg and co-workers found that there[47] was less movement and less respiratory depression in the midazolam–ketamine group than in the methohexitone group, and they did not see postoperative hallucinations. Moscona et al.,[49] on the other hand, did not feel that adding ketamine to midazolam offered any benefit to midazolam alone in sedating patients for rhinoplasty.

More recently ketamine has been combined with propofol and infused continuously. The mixture can be titrated nicely to produce a patient who is very sedated yet breathing spontaneously. In most instances patients are able to maintain normal oxyhaemoglobin saturations whilst breathing room air. The dose varies according to the depth of sedation desired. Badrinath et al.[50] compared four dosage regimens: 1, 2, 3, or 4 mg of ketamine per 10 mg of propofol. An initial bolus of these mixtures calculated to give 300 µg/kg of propofol was followed by a continuous infusion ranging from 50–100 µg/kg/minute of propofol and provided excellent sedation. At the higher doses of ketamine they found more untoward effects (need for airway support, postoperative nausea and vomiting, and pyschotomimetic effects), whilst at the lower doses 'rescue' analgesics were required more frequently. Their findings have been recently confirmed by Mortero et al.[51] It is important to premedicate with midazolam and an anticholinergic, and for longer procedures small doses (0.5–1.0 mg) of midazolam should be given at 30-minute intervals.

Etomidate is most often used for induction of general anaesthesia, but it has been used for sedation.[52] In patients who cannot tolerate even mild degrees of cardiovascular depression it may be helpful, because its use is associated with cardiovascular stability more than any other agent. Unfortunately it has some other characteristics that make it less desirable. Etomidate tends to burn on injection. About a third of the patients exhibit movements mimicking myoclonus, a hazardous effect when performing orbital blocks. Although the movements can be lessened by concomitant administration of either opioids or benzodiazepines, both jeopardize etomidate's cardiovascular stability. It also has a significant incidence of nausea and vomiting, lacks any analgesic effect, and causes adrenal suppression. In the United States the Food and Drug Administration limits continuous infusion of this drug to short procedures due to corticosteroid inhibition.[53]

Antagonists

Because of patient variability in response to predetermined doses of sedatives, relative overdoses will occur. Overdoses of opioids or benzodiazepines can be reversed by the specific antagonists, naloxone and flumazenil, respectively. They should be immediately available whenever these agents are used, with hopes of never having to use them.[40]

Naloxone is a specific μ-opioid antagonist that is devoid of any agonist properties in clinical doses. Divided intravenous doses of 0.1 mg given slowly will rapidly reverse opioid-induced respiratory depression. Normally it should be rare to need more than 0.4 mg to achieve the desired reversal. As the effects last for only 30–45 minutes, additional doses or an infusion may be required should one be dealing with a very large overdose of opioid. Following reversal patients need to be watched carefully as respiratory depression may reoccur. Analgesia, of course, is also reversed, although very careful titration can result in maintenance of analgesia but reversal of respiratory depression. Rapid administration can produce hypertension and tachycardia. Fulminant pulmonary oedema has also been reported following the use of naloxone in a previously healthy young patient.[54]

Flumazenil is a specific benzodiazepine antagonist nearly devoid of any agonist effects, and it reverses all effects. In a patient overly sedated with a benzodiazepine, 0.2–0.4 mg intravenously rapidly results in awakening. As this effect lasts only about 2 hours, re-sedation can occur. Depending on the clinical situation, patients given an overdose of benzodiazepine may need to be observed for prolonged periods of time despite reversal with flumazenil.[55] One must exercise care in giving this agent to people who take benzodiazepines chronically, as withdrawal symptoms, including seizures, may ensue in these patients.[12]

Summary

A summary of the pharmacokinetic and dosage data for the drugs discussed in this chapter can be found in Table 1. The doses given are those recommended for providing sedation only. Titration of dosage must occur due to the variability of response in individual patients and due to possible synergism when multiple agents are used.

The art of providing safe and effective sedation for patients undergoing any surgical procedure is based on knowledge of pharmacokinetics, pharmacodynamics, pathophysiology, and the needs of the patient and surgeon. The following comments summarise many of the points included in this chapter and offer a few additional caveats:

Table 1. Pharmacokinetic and sedative dosage data for commonly used sedatives.

Drug	Redistribution half-life (minutes)	Elimination half-life (hours)	Context-sensitive half-time after 2 hours (minutes)	Bolus dose (70 kg patient)	Infusion rates (μg/kg/min)	Target plasma concentration
Thiopental	3	9	100	12.5–75 mg	*	4–8 μg/ml
Methohexital	5	4	?	5–30 mg	*	1–3 μg/ml
Diazepam	12	40	?	2–3 mg	*	300–400 ng/ml
Midazolam	11	2	45	0.5–2.5 mg	0.25–1.0	40–100 ng/ml
Fentanyl	1.5	4	50	50–100 μg	0.01–0.03	1–2 ng/ml
Sufentanil	1.4	3	20	5–30 μg	0.005–0.01	0.02–0.2 ng/ml
Alfentanil	2	2	50	125–250 μg	0.25–1.0	25–75 ng/ml
Remifentanil	1	9 minutes	3	20–50 μg	0.025–0.1	1.0–2.0 ng/ml
Propofol	3	2	15	10–50 mg	10–50	1–2 μg/ml
Ketamine	14	2	?	10–50 mg	**	0.1–1.0 μg/ml
Etomidate	3	3	?	7–14 mg	7.0	100–300 ng/ml

* These agents are generally not used as continuous infusions in outpatients.
** Ketamine is sometimes combined with propofol as an infusion,[50,51] but rarely infused alone.
Data adapted from a variety of references.[7–12,28,32,34,40]
Values have been rounded for ease of memory and comparison.

- Appropriate monitoring by a trained person is essential to safety. In addition, the person administering sedatives must be aware of their properties and side effects and be able to manage all untoward reactions.
- Thorough knowledge of the patient and the procedure are essential if intelligent choices about the type of sedation and mode of employment are to be made.
- Rapid-acting, short-duration drugs facilitate effective titration without overdosing. This is especially important to the patient who will be going home after day-care surgery.
- In the rare event that antagonists have to be used, the patient must be observed carefully and for sufficient time to ensure that symptoms of overdose do not recur after discharge.
- Using combinations of drugs is rational, helpful, and often necessary. Remember that the possibility of synergism exists when using combinations, and observe patients even more closely.
- Finally, there are no ideal drugs or combination of them.

References

1   Jastak JT, Peskin PM. Major morbidity or mortality from office anesthetic procedures: a closed-claim analysis of 13 cases. *Anesth Prog.* 1991; 38:39–44.
2   American Society of Anesthesiologists. Standards for basic anesthesia monitoring. In: *2001 Directory of Members*. American Society of Anesthesiologists, Park Ridge IL, USA, 2001. pp 493–494.
3   Blouin RT, Seifert HA, Babenco HD, Conard PF, Gross JB. Propofol depresses the hypoxic ventilatory response during conscious sedation and isocapnia. *Anesthesiology.* 1993; 79:1177–1182.
4   Greco RJ, Gonzalez R, Johnson P, Scolieri M, Rekhopf PG, Heckler F. Potential dangers of oxygen supplementation during facial surgery. *Plast Reconstr Surg.* 1995; 95:978–984.
5   Glass PS, Bloom M, Kearse L, Rosow C, Sebel P, Manberg P. Bispectral analysis measures sedation and memory effects of propofol, midazolam, isoflurane, and alfentanil in healthy volunteers. *Anesthesiology.* 1997; 86:836–847.
6   Kearse L, Rosow C, Zaslavsky A, Connors P, Dershwitz M, Denman W. Bispectral analysis of the electroencephalogram predicts conscious processing of information during propofol sedation and hypnosis. *Anesthesiology.* 1998; 88:25–34.
7   Benet LZ, Kroetz DL, Sheiner LB. Pharmacokinetics: the dynamics of drug absorption, distribution, and elimination. In: Hardman JG, Limbird LE, editors. *Goodman and Gilman's the Pharmacological Basis of Therapeutics*, 9th ed. New York, McGraw-Hill, 1996; 3–27.
8   Bürkle H, Dunbar S, Van Aken H. Remifentanil: a novel, short-acting, μ-opioid. *Anesth Analg.* 1996; 83:646–651.
9   Greenberg CP, DeSoto H. Sedation techniques. In: Twersky RS, editor. *The Ambulatory Anesthesia Handbook*. St. Louis, Mosby Year Book, 1995. pp 301–359.
10   Hughes MA, Glass PSA, Jacobs JR. Context-sensitive half-time in multicompartment pharmacokinetic models for intravenous anesthetic drugs. *Anesthesiology.* 1992; 76:334–341.

11   Kapila A, Glass PSA, Jacobs JR, Muir KT, Hermann DJ, Shiraishi M, Howell S, Smith RL. Measured context-sensitive half-times of remifentanil and alfentanil. *Anesthesiology*. 1995; 83:968–975.

12   Hobbs WR, Rall TW, Verdoorn TA. Hypnotics and sedatives; ethanol. In: Hardman JG, Limbird LE, editors. *Goodman and Gilman's the Pharmacological Basis of Therapeutics*, 9th ed. New York, McGraw-Hill, 1996. pp 361–396.

13   Bovill JG. Mechanisms of intravenous anesthesia. In: White PF, editor. *Intravenous Anesthesia*. Williams & Wilkins, Baltimore, 1997. pp 27–46.

14   Short TG, Plummer JL, Chui PT. Hypnotic and anaesthetic interactions between midazolam, propofol, and alfentanil. *Br J Anaesth*. 1992. pp 162–167.

15   Bailey PL, Pace NL, Ashburn MA, Moll JW, East KA, Stanley TH. Frequent hypoxemia and apnea after sedation with midazolam and fentanyl. *Anesthesiology*. 1990; 73:826–830.

16   Mertens MJ, Vuyk J, Olofsen E, Bovill JG, Burm AGL. Propofol alters the pharmacokinetics of alfentanil in healthy male volunteers. *Anesthesiology*. 2001; 94:949–957.

17   Vinik HR. Intravenous anaesthetic drug interactions: practical applications. *Eur J Anaesthesiol*. 1995; 12 (suppl. 12):13–19.

18   Vinik HR. Intravenous drug interactions in anesthesia and their clinical implications. *Am J Anesthesiol* 1996; 23 (Suppl S1):9–14.

19   Epstein RH, Mendel HG, Witkowski TA, Waters R, Guarniari KM, Marr AT, Lessin JB. The safety and efficacy of oral transmucosal fentanyl citrate for preoperative sedation in young children. *Anesth Analg*. 1996; 83:1200–1205.

20   Egan TD, Sharma A, Ashburn MA, Kievit J, Pace NL, Streisand JB. Multiple dose pharmacokinetics of oral transmucosal fentanyl citrate in healthy volunteers. *Anesthesiology*. 2000; 92:665–673.

21   Struys M, Versichelen L, Rolly G. Influence of pre-anaesthetic medication on target propofol concentration using a 'Diprifusor' TCI system during ambulatory surgery. *Anaesthesia*. 1998; 53 (Suppl):68–71.

22   Janzen PR, Hall WJ, Hopkins PM. Setting targets for sedation with a target-controlled propofol infusion. *Anaesthesia*. 2000; 55:666–669.

23   Struys MM, DeSmet T, Depoorter B, Versichelen LF, Mortier EP, Dumortier FJ, Shafer SL, Rolly G. Comparison of plasma compartment versus two methods for effect compartment-controlled target-controlled infusion for propofol. *Anesthesiology*. 2000; 92:399–406.

24   Pac-Soo CK, Deacock S, Lockwood G, Carr C, Whitwam JG. Patient-controlled sedation for cataract surgery using peribulbar block. *Br J Anaesth*. 1996; 77:370–374.

25   Janzen PRM, Christys A, Vucevic M. Patient-controlled sedation using propofol in elderly patients in day-case cataract surgery. *Br J Anaesth*. 1999; 82:635–636.

26   Herrick IA, Gelb AW, Nichols B, Kirby J. Patient-controlled propofol sedation for elderly patients: safety and patient attitude toward control. *Can J Anaesth*. 1996; 43:1014–1018.

27   Kitagawa E, Iida A, Kimura Y, Kumagai M, Nakamura M, Kamekura N, Fujisawa T, Fukushima K. Response to intravenous sedation by elderly patients at the Hokkaido University Dental Hospital. *Anesth Prog*. 1992; 39:73–78.

28   Philip BK. Pharmacology of intravenous sedative agents. In: Rogers MC, Tinker JH, Covino BG, Longnecker DE, editors. *Principles and Practice of Anesthesiology*. Mosby Year Book, St. Louis, 1993. pp 1087–1104.

29   Parikh SS, Chung F. Postoperative delirium in the elderly. *Anesth Analg*. 1995; 80:1223–1232.

30   Rasmussen L, Steentoft A, Rasmussen H, Kristensen P, Moller J, the ISPOC group. Benzodiazepines and postoperative cognitive dysfunction in the elderly. *Br J Anaesth*. 1999; 83:585–589.

31   Fredman B, Lahav M, Zohar E, Golod M, Paruta I, Jedeikin R. The effect of
      midazolam premedication on mental and psychomotor recovery in geriatric patients
      undergoing brief surgical procedures. *Anesth Analg.* 1999; 89:1161–1166.

32   Benet LZ, Øie S, Schwartz JB. Design and optimization of dosage regimens: phar-
      macologic data. In: Hardman JG, Limbird LE, editors. *Goodman and Gilman's the
      Pharmacological Basis of Therapeutics*, 9th ed. New York, McGraw-Hill, 1996.
      pp 1707–1792.

33   Rosow CE, Dershwitz M. Pharmacology of opioid analgesic agents. In: Longnecker
      DE, Tinker JH, Morgan GE, Jr., editors. *Principles and Practice of Anesthesiology.*
      Mosby Year Book, St. Louis, 1993. pp 1233–1259.

34   Reisine T, Pasternak G. Opioid analgesics and antagonists. In: Hardman JG, Limbird
      LE, editors. *Goodman and Gilman's the Pharmacological Basis of Therapeutics*, 9th
      ed. New York, McGraw-Hill, 1996. pp 521–555.

35   Grond S, Lynch J, Diefenbach C, Altrock K, Lehmann KA. Comparison of
      ondansetron and droperidol in the prevention of nausea and vomiting after inpatient
      minor gynecologic surgery. *Anesth Analg.* 1995; 81:603–607.

36   Burns TA, Shomaker TS, Patel BCK, Crandall A, Pace NL, Kern SE, Satovick NJ,
      Meyfroidt GJP. Comparison of oral transmucosal fentanyl citrate and intravenous fen-
      tanyl citrate for perioperative sedation/analgesia for cataract surgery. *Am J Anesthe-
      siol.* 2001; 28:35–39.

37   Yee JB, Schafer PG, Crandall AS, Pace NL. Comparison of methohexital and alfen-
      tanil on movement during placement of retrobulbar nerve block. *Anesth Analg.* 1994;
      79:320–323.

38   Langevin S, Lessard MR, Trépanier CA, Baribault J. Alfentanil causes less post-
      operative nausea and vomiting than equipotent doses of fentanyl or sufentanil in out-
      patients. *Anesthesiology.* 1999; 91:1666–1673.

39   Glass PSA, Gan TJ, Howell S. A review of the pharmacokinetics and pharmaco-
      dynamics of remifentanil. *Anesth Analg.* 1999; 89(Suppl):S7–S14.

40   Fanning GL. Sedation Techniques. In: Davis DB, Mandel MR, editors. *Ophthalmol-
      ogy Clinics of North America.* WB Saunders Co., Philadelphia, 1998; 73–85.

41   Neel S, Deitch R Jr., Moorthy SS, Dierdorf S, Yee R. Changes in intraocular pressure
      during low-dose intravenous sedation with propofol before cataract surgery. *Br J Oph-
      thalmol.* 1995; 70:1093–1097.

42   Ferrari LR, Donlon JV. A comparison of propofol, midazolam, and methohexital for
      sedation during retrobulbar and peribulbar block. *J Clin Anesth.* 1992; 4:93–96.

43   Raeder JC, Misvaer G. Comparison of propofol induction with thiopentone or metho-
      hexitone in short outpatient general anaesthesia. *Acta Anaesthesiol Scand.* 1988;
      32:607–613.

44   Tang J, Chen L. White PF, Watcha MF, Wender RH, Naruse R, Kariger R, Sloninsky
      A. Recovery profile, costs, and patient satisfaction with propofol and sevoflurane for
      fast-track office-based anesthesia. *Anesthesiology.* 1999; 91:253–261.

45   Stead SW, Beatie CD, Keyes MA. Anesthesia for ophthalmic surgery. In: Longnecker
      DE, Tinker JK, Morgan GE Jr., editors. *Principles and Practice of Anesthesiology.*
      Mosby Year Book, St. Louis, 1993. pp 2181–2199.

46   Vinnik CA. An intravenous dissociation technique for outpatient plastic surgery: tran-
      quility in the office surgical facility. *Plast Reconstr Surg.* 1981; 67:799–805.

47   Rosenberg MK, Raymond C, Bridge PD. Comparison of midazolam/ketamine with
      methohexital for sedation during peribulbar block. *Anesth Analg.* 1995; 81:173–174.

48   White PF, Vasconez LO, Mathes SA, Way WL, Wender LA. Comparison of midazo-
      lam and diazepam sedation during plastic surgery. *Plast Reconstr Surg.* 1988;
      81:703–712.

49   Moscona RA, Ramon I, Ben-David B, Isserles S. A comparison of sedation techniques for outpatient rhinoplasty: midazolam versus midazolam plus ketamine. *Plast Reconstr Surg.* 1995; 96:1066–1074.

50   Badrinath S, Avramov MN, Shadrick M, Witt TR, Ivankovich AD. The use of ketamine-propofol combination during monitored anesthesia care. *Anesth Analg.* 2000; 90:858–862.

51   Mortero RF, Clark LD, Tolan MM, Metz RJ, Tsueda K, Sheppard RA. The effects of small-dose ketamine on propofol sedation: respiration, postoperative mood, perception, cognition, and pain. *Anesth Analg.* 2001; 92:1465–1469.

52   Urquhart ML, White PF. Comparison of sedative infusions during regional anesthesia-methohexital, etomidate, and midazolam. *Anesth Analg.* 1989; 68:249–254.

53   Gupta VL, Glass PSA. Total Intravenous Anesthesia. In: Longnecker DE, Tinker JH, Morgan GE Jr., editors. *Principles and Practice of Anesthesiology.* Mosby Year Book, St. Louis, 1993. pp 1260–1293.

54   André RA. Sudden death following naloxone administration. *Anesth Analg.* 1980; 59:782–784.

55   Ghouri AF, Ramirez Ruiz MA, White PF. Effect of flumazenil on recovery after midazolam and propofol sedation. *Anesthesiology* 1994; 81:333–339.

9

High-Volume Cataract Surgery

Mr Jerry Hill, CRNA
Miss Gina Stancel, CST, COA, HCRM

Introduction

The definition of high-volume cataract surgery is variable, changing in relation to the locality and the care providers. In a small community, a practice doing a thousand cataract procedures a year would be considered high-volume, whilst a few surgeons in the United States perform more than 5000 per year each. Perhaps more important than the absolute volume of cases completed is the rate at which they are performed. If 5000 cases are performed in 2000 hours (2.5 cases per hour), the logistical needs of the anaesthesia and surgical teams are entirely different from the requirements of those doing the same number of cases in 500 hours (10 cases per hour). For the purposes of this chapter, we will choose the latter rate as the definition of a high-volume practice, although in our centre we occasionally maintain a pace of 15 uncomplicated cataract procedures per hour for up to three hours for a single surgeon.

Quality care is the primary goal of every facility. An additional important goal is efficiency. This is especially true in the United States, where shrinking reimbursements and rising costs are challenging the very existence of many institutions. Thus, whilst one must never compromise quality for speed, one should also recognise that efficiency is an integral part of high quality. A skilful surgeon operating quickly has an opportunity to minimise surgical trauma and to reduce the incidence of inflammation.[1,2] Shorter operations allow us to use short-acting local anaesthetics and sedatives, resulting in a rapid recovery time and a speedy return to normal activities for the patient. Quickly moving through a well-organised system also gives the patient less time to become anxious and fidgety, reducing the need for sedatives and anxiolytics.

In a system providing quality care at a high-volume rate, the anaesthesia team is only one part of an entire spectrum of caregivers who are responsible for the total surgical output. Anaesthetists can only care for patients at the rate they can be admitted and prepared. Likewise, surgeons cannot operate faster than patients and operating rooms can be prepared for them. In our facility, a well-trained crew endeavours to keep the surgeon working at maximum efficiency, which means no down time between patients. Thus, if the surgeon can do a cataract procedure in six minutes, then the total output should be 10 cases per hour. This is best accomplished with adequate staff working with two operating rooms; however, even with one operating room, the turnover time can be reduced to two minutes.

The purpose of this chapter is to describe how quality care is achieved at a high-volume rate in our facility. As noted, quality care is a multi-factorial process with anaesthesia being but one part. If our method is to be emulated successfully, all of the parts must be examined and implemented. Whilst reading, it will be useful to keep in mind the three key elements that apply to every part of the system: consistency, simplicity, and reproducibility.

The Facility

It is not necessary to have an elaborate facility to perform high-quality, high-volume surgery. The surgical facility at the Eye Centers of Florida is neither large nor opulent. Patients initially arrive in the reception area, which seats 30. In the preoperative holding area there are six cubicles separated by curtains. We have eight stretchers, one for each cubicle and one for each operating theatre. There are two operating theatres separated by a sub-sterile area containing three autoclaves. The small recovery room contains only chairs for the patients to sit on whilst eating a small meal prior to discharge. The only other spaces in the facility are offices, record room, and supply storage.

Patient Referrals

Patients enter the system in several ways (see Appendix 1). Some are established patients within our system, whilst optometrists, family physicians, or friends refer others. Because of our location in a resort area, some patients have had their cataracts diagnosed by their physicians at home but choose to have surgery at our facility during their stay in Florida over the winter.

Patients referred by physicians or optometrists who have already been diagnosed as having a cataract causing visual dysfunction are scheduled to see the surgeon in the morning so that surgery can be performed in the afternoon. The patients are informed ahead of time that they might have surgery on the same day, which allows them to come prepared. Many have seen the preoperative instruction packets that are available in satellite offices. Others are given instructions by phone when making an appointment.

The surgeon sees the patient before any other testing or counselling is performed. This is necessary both for confirmation of the diagnosis and for initiating the appropriate orders for the proposed surgery. If surgery is to be performed, the patient sees a counsellor who discusses the procedure, obtains consent, and takes the patient to the admitting department, which is located in the main clinic. Having the final cataract evaluation and surgery on the same day is very appealing to many patients, as it saves them an extra trip and allows them to have their corrective surgery as soon as possible.

The Admitting Process

In our admitting department in the clinical area there are two registered nurses and a physician's assistant who perform the preoperative history and physical examinations. When deemed necessary, the patient's family physician is consulted if further evaluation and clearance is required. Technicians are available here who perform any testing that may be required as determined by the history and physical examinations, as well as all the preoperative eye testing and measurements for calculation of the intraocular lens. The patient may remain in the admitting department for 30–45 minutes. During this time the written consent for surgery is obtained, perioperative orders are reviewed and completed, postoperative prescriptions are written, and postoperative instructions are given. Accomplishing all of these tasks before the patient arrives in the surgery centre saves a great deal of time, especially in the recovery room.

Foreseeing and preventing problems is essential in maintaining an uninterrupted flow of patients. If a problem surfaces after the patient reaches the anaesthetist, there will be a delay; therefore, problems must be recognised or ruled out before the patient progresses very far into the system. Having our patients screened by a physician's assistant and/or nurse practitioner has been very beneficial in preventing delays. The anaesthesia and admitting departments have worked diligently to establish protocols for dealing with a variety of circumstances that may be revealed by the history and physical examinations: diabetes, hypertension, coagulation defects, the need for more thorough medical evaluation, and so forth. Using protocols (see Appendix 2 and Chapter 5) allows rapid triaging and/or management of patients with minimal waiting. If an unusual problem occurs, the anaesthesia and admitting teams formally discuss it later in order to determine if it could have been foreseen and resolved. Having the patient thoroughly screened and prepared allows the anaesthetist to proceed without interruption.[3]

In our hands, high-volume cataract surgery is best performed in the afternoon. It allows us to have adequate time for the admitting process and permits us to have an open-ended schedule. The surgeons often see patients in the morning and add them to that afternoon's list if there is room; thus, patients are often scheduled right up to the beginning of the day's surgery. Longer surgeries or cases with anticipated difficulties are scheduled at the end of the list in order to prevent backups in the waiting and preparation areas.

Arriving in the Surgery Centre

On arrival in the centre, a receptionist receives the patient, verifies that the consent has been signed, and organises the paperwork. The clinic chart accompanies the patient, but a separate chart is initiated in the surgery centre. A technician sees the patient next, reviews the history and physical, and instils the dilating drops. The technician then accompanies the patients to the preoperative holding area and assists them onto the stretcher. Patients are not required to change clothing. Family members are required to remain in the reception area. The technician is responsible for alerting the anaesthetist of anything unusual about the patient at this point. The patient is now given over to a nurse, who checks all the paperwork and reviews the history and physical examination again. This nurse also reviews the intraocular lens calculations and assures that the correct lens is available to accompany the patient. A nurse or technician pulls all of the lenses for the day from the storage room prior to the start of the surgical list. If there is anything unusual about the patient, this nurse insures that the anaesthetist has been informed.

Adequate staffing is absolutely essential to maintain a flow of one patient every four to five minutes. In times of greatest need, assistants from the clinical area come to the surgery centre. There are nine people participating in patient care from the reception area to, but not including, the operating room. Most of the staff have been cross-trained in order to fill multiple positions whenever necessary, such as during staff absences.

Anaesthesia

There are two anaesthetists at our institution, one to perform the block and the other to monitor the patient in the operating room, and they alternate functions weekly. When the patient arrives in the preparation area, the anaesthetist reviews the history and physical examination and any laboratory work that might have been done, confirms that the permit has been signed, and notes the vital signs and the axial length of the globe. Intravenous access is achieved, and a self-sealing injection port is attached to the catheter. Topical anaesthetic drops are applied to the operative eye and a small dose of sedative (i.e., 1–3 mg midazolam) is administered. Whilst the sedative is taking effect, the anaesthetist goes to the next patient and repeats all of the above steps. On returning to the sedated patient, the anaesthetist performs a modified retrobulbar block using an inferotemporal transconjunctival approach with a 1 ¼" needle as previously described,[4,5] after which an ocular compression device is applied. The anaesthetist then goes back to the second patient, who has already been examined and sedated, and performs the block. The process is then repeated until all of the patients have been prepared.

A registered nurse is designated as an anaesthesia assistant. This person obtains an ECG rhythm strip, instils eye drops, and assists in starting the intravenous and administering the block. As we may delegate other tasks to this person, such as administering other drugs, we prefer that he/she be a nurse. A technician follows the patient after the block, checking the vital signs and noting the degree of akinesia some 8–10 minutes after the block. Blocks are not supplemented unless there is total failure to achieve akinesia in more than one extraocular muscle or marked orbicularis function.

Topical anaesthesia has been tried in our institution and has been used quite successfully in many others.[6] We feel that the modified retrobulbar block works very well for us by eliminating some intraoperative steps, by providing an akinetic eye, and by allowing the surgeon to concentrate totally on the surgical procedure. Morbidity rates are extremely small using either anaesthetic technique,[7,8] but we feel that the block makes the experience more acceptable to everyone, including both surgeons and patients.

The Operating Theatre

There are six staff members assigned to the two operating theatres in the facility. Each theatre has a circulating nurse and a scrub technician who remain in the room until the list is completed. The remaining two staff members are responsible for moving the patients in and out of the theatres and for maintaining the instruments.

For the system to work efficiently, there must be enough instruments and supplies. Custom-prepared packs containing all of the disposable supplies required by the surgeon are helpful both for efficiency and cost containment. These packs should be organized to facilitate quick opening and use with minimal handling. Each theatre has a rolling cart stocked with custom packs, extra equipment, and other supplies so that the nurse never has to leave the room. Instrumentation is standardized in each theatre using interchangeable instrument trays. Having five such trays and three autoclaves allows us to keep pace with the surgeon. There are only eight instruments on each tray: a lid speculum, a diamond knife, a forceps, a 23G bent needle, a phacoemulsification handpiece, a Bechert nucleus rotator, an I/A handpiece, and an IOL injector. Extra sterile instruments are available in each theatre. A technician is assigned to clean and re-sterilise instruments between cases.

The patient is transported to the operating theatre on a stretcher by a technician, who performs the surgical prep. The scrub technician drapes the patient whilst the circulating nurse prepares the phacoemulsification machine and the microscope. The surgeon performs surgery in the same way, using the fewest possible steps in each case. This consistency and reproducibility promotes staff efficiency, because they are able to anticipate every step. The surgeon and the staff work continuously without delays until the lists are completed. If everyone on the team remains utterly dedicated to the task, a rate of 10 or more procedures per hour can be consistently achieved.

We have found it unnecessary to follow some of the time-honoured but time-consuming practices of the past. It is not necessary to completely mop the floor of the theatre between each patient nor is it necessary to do a complete hand scrub each time. We have had no increase in infections or other complications by eliminating these steps. We are constantly looking for other ways to safely save time, examining every step of our process.

Recovery

At the end of the procedure, the technician responsible for transporting patients instils the postoperative drops, removes the drape, and takes the patient to the recovery room. No eye patch is applied. The patients are told to begin using their postoperative eye drops when they are able to start opening and closing the eyelid. Once out of the theatre, the patient's vital signs are obtained once more and the intravenous is removed. The patient then walks the short distance to the recovery area to receive a small meal prior to discharge. The postoperative instructions and appointment time for the first postoperative visit are reviewed at this time. Patients are also given a packet of material containing general information, emergency contact numbers, written postoperative instructions, and a patient-satisfaction questionnaire. The latter is used in our continuing quality assurance process. In general, patients are in the surgical facility for less than an hour.

In summary, several issues should be emphasised:

- Whilst adequate numbers of supplies and staff are essential in a high-volume practice, elaborate facilities are not.
- Given a trained, dedicated staff and two operating rooms, a surgeon can operate non-stop until finished with the list.
- Whenever possible, sacred cows should be eliminated, such as completely mopping the floors and doing full hand scrubbing between cases.
- Staff who are not completely committed to providing quality care with maximum efficiency are not tolerated.
- Afternoon surgery allows for an open-ended list, which facilitates late scheduling and even 'same-day' surgery.
- The surgeon must be as committed to efficiency as the staff. Stopping unnecessarily between cases for any reason demoralizes the members of the staff who have been working hard to achieve the maximum turnover rate.
- Good care should never be compromised for the sake of speed. On the other hand, efficiency and quality do more than co-exist—they are complimentary.
- Finally, the most important elements in a successful high-volume practice are consistency, simplicity, and reproducibility.

References

1   Fujishima H, Toda I, Yagi Y, Tsubota K. Quantitative evaluation of postsurgical inflammation by infrared radiation thermometer and laser flare-cell meter. *J Cataract Refract Surg.* 1994; 20:451–454.
2   Mueller-Jensen K, Rorig M, Hagele J, Zimmermann H. Effect of cataract technique and duration of surgery on fibrin reaction after IOL implantation. *Ophthalmologe.* 1997; 94:38–40.

3   Fischer SP. Development and effectiveness of an anesthesia preoperative evaluation clinic in a teaching hospital. *Anesthesiology.* 1996; 85:196–206.

4   Hamilton RC, Loken RG. Modified retrobulbar block. *Can J Anaesth.* 1993; 40:1219–1220.

5   Hustead RF, Hamilton RC, Loken RG. Periocular local anesthesia: medial orbital as an alternative to superior nasal injection. *J Cataract Refract Surg.* 1994; 20:197–201.

6   Shammas HJ, Milkie M, Yeo R. Topical and subconjunctival anesthesia for phaco-emulsification: prospective study. *J Cataract Refract Surg.* 1997; 23:1577–1580.

7   Boezaart A, Berry R, Nell M. Topical anesthesia versus retrobulbar block for cataract surgery: the patients' perspective. *J Clin Anesth.* 2000; 12:58–60.

8   Jacobi PC, Dietlein TS, Jacobi FK. A comparative study of topical vs retrobulbar anesthesia in complicated cataract surgery. *Arch Ophthalmol.* 2000; 118:1037–1043.

Appendix 1. Patient Flow Chart

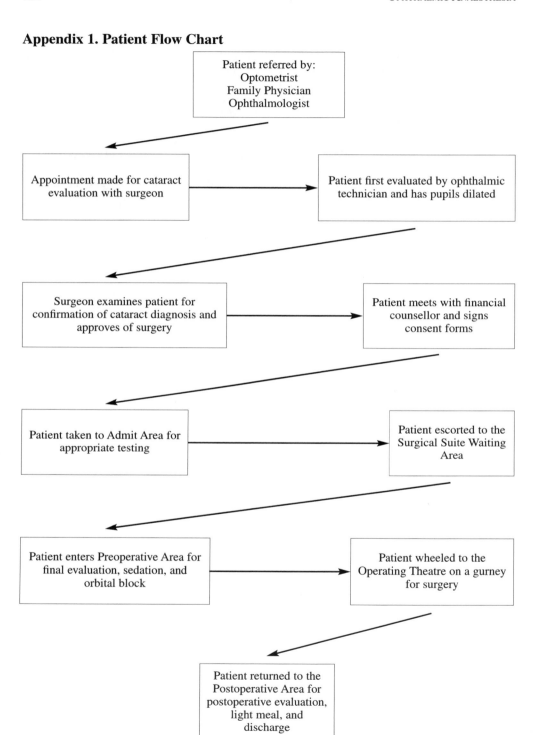

Appendix 2. Eye Centers of Florida/Surgicare Preoperative Testing Protocols for Cataract Surgery

Objective

To review the physical and mental status of the patient prior to ophthalmic surgery to determine that proper documentation is available and/or noted discrepancies resolved.

Policy

To provide quality patient care and adhere to guidelines regarding medical testing. All patients will be individually assessed and preoperative testing ordered as deemed necessary.

Procedure

A. Hypertension

Patients presenting with a systolic blood pressure reading above 180 mm Hg or a diastolic blood pressure reading above 90 mm Hg, will be evaluated by the nurse clinician with consultation with the anaesthesia provider and/or attending surgeon. Intervention will be initiated as deemed appropriate with follow-up to the patient's referring physician as deemed appropriate.

B. Temperature

Patients presenting with an oral/auditory temperature above 102 degrees F, or below 93 degrees F, will require consultation with the anesthesia provider and/or attending surgeon prior to any scheduled surgery.

C. Pulse

Patients presenting with a sustained pulse rate above 100/min or below 50/min accompanied with ECG changes, will be reviewed by the anaesthesia provider and/or attending surgeon. Exceptions will be those patients with a known pre-existing bradycardia, or those patients presently taking a prescribed beta-blocker. In those cases the unacceptable pulse rate would be 45/min.

D. Diuretics

1. Patients will be required to indicate if they have a history of low potassium. They will be evaluated for evidence of abnormality related to fluid and electrolyte imbalance, i.e. poor skin turgor, ECG abnormality, or dehydration.
2. Patients presenting with a serum potassium below 3.5 mEq/l or above 5.7 mEq/l, will require consultation with the anaesthesia provider and/or attending surgeons to determine proper management.
3. Symptomatic patients will be brought to the attention of the anaesthesia provider and/or attending surgeon to determine appropriate care or consultation.

E. Diabetic Patients

Patients presenting with a blood sugar below 70 mg/dl or above 400 mg/dl will require consultation with the anaesthesia provider and/or attending surgeon and intervention initiated as the standard of care dictates. A follow-up with the patient's referring physician will occur if deemed necessary.

F. Electrocardiogram

Patients presenting with an abnormal ECG will be evaluated by the nurse clinician and anaesthesia provider prior to surgery. The attending surgeon will be consulted if necessary.

G. Prior Hospitalisation/Treatment

Any patient hospitalised for a CVA, an acute MI, or having a cardiac catheterisation or cardiac angioplasty within 90 days of the planned surgery will require medical release from the attending physician. Patients scheduled for surgery after 90 days from the aforementioned events will be assessed on an individual basis and medical clearance obtained if the condition warrants.

10

Anaesthesia for Paediatric Ophthalmological Surgery

Dr Chandra M. Kumar
Prof Chris Dodds

Introduction

This chapter will deal with the basic conduct of anaesthesia for the common ophthalmic procedures performed in children. The readers are encouraged to read other chapters in this book and other textbooks of paediatric anaesthesia for further knowledge.

The paediatric patient may present for a variety of ophthalmological procedures ranging from a simple day case to the more complicated procedures requiring hospital admission. The commonest planned paediatric operations undertaken are:

- Strabismus correction;
- probing for congenital nasolacrimal duct obstruction;
- congenital cataract extractions;
- congenital ptosis.

Less common but important reasons for presentation for ophthalmic operations in children are:

- Infantile glaucoma;
- ocular tumours;
- laser therapy for retinopathy of prematurity in neonates has become a common undertaking;
- trauma and perforating eye injuries form the commonest unplanned procedures.

The anaesthetic management of children demands a basic understanding of age-related changes in anatomy, physiology, and pharmacology. The preoperative assessment and conduct of anaesthesia can then be tailored to meet the particular

needs of the surgical procedure and postoperative care. Age will affect the anaesthetic management, because the patient may be a premature infant or a mature
teenager. Additionally, paediatric patients vary from those with no other medical
problems to those with very complicated medical problems, rare syndromes, or a
predisposition to malignant hyperpyrexia (MH).

Although simple procedures, such as nasolacrimal duct probing and irrigation, may
be carried out in small hospitals, the more complicated procedures are usually dealt
with in big centres by experienced anaesthetists. There is no single technique that can
be advocated for all procedures. Although the practice of anaesthesia varies from centre to centre, they are all founded on the basic principles of paediatric anaesthesia.

Anatomy

For anaesthetists, the most important anatomical differences in children relate to the
airways. They have narrow nasal passages, yet neonates are obligate nose breathers
until later in development, usually after three months of age. The larynx is anteriorly
placed and the narrowest part of the conducting airway is at the cricoid ring. The tra-
chea is short and the mainstem bronchi bifurcate at equal angles, predisposing to
endobronchial intubation on either side. Intubation may be difficult in children
because of their relatively large heads and short, floppy necks. The tongue is often
pushed against the palate, causing respiratory obstruction during induction of anaesthesia. Small amounts of mucus may also cause considerable airway obstruction.
Some of the more complex syndromes affecting the orbit, especially mass lesions,
may also compromise the airway.

Physiology

In infants the respiratory muscles tire easily and immature alveoli are prone to collapse making gaseous exchange less efficient. Respiratory control systems are not
fully developed until after 6 months of age, which can result in periodic apnoea that
may be more pronounced during or after general anaesthesia. The myocardium is
immature and has limited contractility leading to a relatively fixed stroke volume, so
that cardiac output is largely determined by the heart rate. Anaesthetic agents may
have depressant effects on the myocardium and may further reduce oxygen delivery,
which is especially important in young children who have a relatively high oxygen
consumption. Indeed, neonates have approximately twice the metabolic rate of
adults, largely to fuel growth and for thermoregulation. During the first year of life,
renal function has not developed its maximum efficiency and electrolyte and/or fluid
imbalance will not be well tolerated.

Intraocular Pressure
Normally intraocular pressure (IOP) ranges from 10 to 20 mm Hg (see Chapter 3),
and autoregulatory mechanisms control sudden rises in IOP. A sudden increase in

IOP can precipitate acute glaucoma and cause visual damage. If the globe is open, an increase in IOP can result in loss of vitreous, lens prolapse, or haemorrhage. Hence control of IOP is a major consideration during intraocular surgery.

Factors Affecting IOP in Children

Any rise in venous pressure, such as occurs during crying, may increase the IOP. The anaesthetic drugs used for induction and maintenance are central nervous system depressants and generally lower the IOP,[1–6] although ketamine causes the extraocular muscles to contract and may raise the IOP[7]. If laryngoscopy and endotracheal intubation are performed with inadequate anaesthesia they may also increase the IOP.[6,8] Non-depolarising neuromuscular blocking agents do not have significant effects on the IOP[9–13] but suxamethonium produces a brief rise of about 7 mm Hg.[14,15] This increase is transient and has little consequence in normal patients but if IOP is already raised or if the globe is open, this may have deleterious effects.

Oculo-cardiac Reflex

The oculo-cardiac reflex (see Chapter 3) is a phenomenon usually manifested by bradycardia, cardiac standstill, or dysrhythmias, both atrial and ventricular. It is seen during many paediatric ophthalmological procedures. The afferent limb of the reflex arc is carried by the trigeminal nerve and the efferent limb by the vagus. The incidence of the oculo-cardiac reflex is high and largely depends on age or type of surgery.[16,17] The reflex more frequently occurs in younger children during orbital or strabismus surgery, especially during muscle traction. There are many approaches to the management of this reflex but their efficacy is controversial. If the reflex is observed during strabismus surgery, the surgeon is told to immediately release the traction on the muscle. If the reflex still occurs after another pull, an anticholinergic drug (atropine 10–20 μg kg^{-1} or glycopyrrolate 10 μg kg^{-1}) can be given intravenously.[18] Glycopyrrolate may be less likely to result in the excess tachycardia and tachyarrhythmias frequently seen following atropine administration under general anaesthesia.[18] Many anaesthetists prefer to administer an anticholinergic agent before surgery begins in the paediatric age group.

Pharmacology

The response to administered drugs changes throughout development because of alterations in pharmacokinetics and pharmacodynamics.[19] Both of these parameters can change independently and make it more difficult to predict drug effects in paediatric patients. For example, propofol dosage requirements for both induction and maintenance may be twice as great for a small child as for an adult, with older children and teenagers falling in between. Minimum Alveolar Concentration (MAC) for sevoflurane is also considerably greater in the young.[20]

Anaesthetic Management

Preoperative Evaluation

Anaesthetic management may be affected by many factors. These include the patient, the expertise of the anaesthetist, the proposed operation, and the expertise of the surgeon. A general history, including family, medical, surgical, drug, and allergy, should be taken and appropriate physical examinations performed. A recent history of upper respiratory tract infection is important because these patients are more likely to desaturate in the intraoperative and postoperative periods and to have irritable airways.[21]

Infants with the retinopathy of prematurity (ROP) may suffer from multiple disorders. These include respiratory dysfunction (broncho-pulmonary dysplasia), cardiovascular problems (bradycardia, patent ductus arteriosus, tetralogy of Fallot, and others), neurological problems (intraventricular haemorrhage, hydrocephalus, myelomeningocele), and other more uncommon problems such as subglottic stenosis.[22]

Congenital cataracts may occur in infants with inborn errors of metabolism or intrauterine infection, hence a clear parental history is important. Investigations are ordered depending on concurrent diseases.[22]

Preoperative Instructions

Parents must be instructed to follow the local fasting guidelines both for liquids and solids. Parents may be tempted to console the child by giving sweets or drinks when they are upset, thirsty or hungry. Children are more likely to regurgitate and aspirate because they have a lower gastric pH and greater residual volumes after fasting compared to adults. Longer periods of preoperative fasting may cause discomfort, dehydration and metabolic upset in younger children. Fasting regimens vary[23–25] but solids should be withheld for four (breast milk) to six hours whilst clear liquids may be allowed until 2–3 hours prior to the time of surgery.

Premedication

Many surgical procedures are done as a day case and time may not be available to administer premedication, although it may be required in complicated cases. Premedication is administered to decrease the child's anxiety, facilitate separation between parents and child, decrease anaesthetic requirement during induction, and reduce postoperative nausea and vomiting. If premedication is required, the choice and route of premedication is determined by the preferences of the anaesthetist. Heavy premedication may be undesirable. If sedation is required, benzodiazepines or antihistmines are preferable to opioids, due to the opioids propensity for causing nausea and vomiting. The use of topical local anaesthetic creams, such as EMLA cream, has made intravenous access easier. The use of anticholinergic agents as premedication has largely vanished except in rare instances where the prediction of a difficult airway is anticipated and in the very young (<6 months) in whom unwanted parasympathetic effects are common. Premedication can be given by a number of routes such as oral, nasal, or rectal, but injections are best avoided if possible. Some medications may also be administered for surgical reasons, such as mydiatric eye drops for patients undergoing examination under anaesthesia. Mydiatric eye drops may not be tolerated by the child when awake and some delay will be inevitable to allow the drops to be effective.

General Considerations During Anaesthesia

The basic principles and goals of anaesthesia are the same for adults and children. Parental presence in the anaesthetic room is a matter of the discretion of anaesthetist. Whilst of little importance to the child, it probably improves the parents' perception of the surgical experience. If parents are allowed to witness induction, they must be well informed in advance what they are likely to see. They must also agree to leave the room immediately if asked to do so. The presence of parents may be undesirable if they are upset and disruptive prior to induction, or if a difficult induction is expected. The help of a skilled assistant is essential, and as much monitoring as possible should be connected to the patient prior to induction. Pulse oximetry is usually well tolerated.

Induction

The choice between the intravenous and inhalational induction lies with the anaesthetist and the disposition of the child. Much depends on the age of the patient and the ability of the anaesthetist to secure an intravenous cannula, especially in small children. Prepubertal children generally choose an inhalation induction when given a choice, whilst older children frequently agree to an intravenous induction. Gas induction with sevoflurane has largely replaced halothane, due to its more pleasant odour, absence of adverse airway phenomena, and speed. Once an appropriate level of anaesthesia is obtained, venous access is obtained, and the airway is secured using either a laryngeal mask airway or an endotracheal tube.

If intravenous access is easily achieved preoperatively, one may choose to perform an intravenous induction, using propofol 2–3 mg kg^{-1}, for instance. Induction doses tend to be larger, relative to body weight, for children than adults, as previously mentioned.[26] Propofol is associated with significantly less postoperative nausea and vomiting than thiopentone and is associated with a very pleasant recovery from anaesthesia.[27] Neuromuscular blocking agents may be given to facilitate endotracheal tube insertion. An anticholinergic agent may be administered on induction to prevent the oculo-cardiac reflex and to prevent the parasympathetically mediated events (bradycardia, apnoea, mucorrhea) seen in younger infants.[22]

Endotracheal Intubation vs Laryngeal Mask Airway (LMA)

Most anaesthetists prefer to secure the airway with an endotracheal tube but this necessitates the use of muscle relaxants and subsequent reversal. Laryngoscopy and endotracheal intubation are associated with an increased heart rate and a slight increase in the IOP.[6,8] The duration of muscle relaxation may be longer than the expected duration of surgery if reversal is not administered. The LMA is widely used in ophthalmic practice because it does not restrict the surgical access, avoids the use of muscle relaxants, and is less stimulating to the cardiovascular system.[28] However, the LMA does not protect the airway against acid aspiration. The mask may be improperly positioned and may also shift after placement causing partial airway obstruction. Many anaesthetists are reluctant to use the LMA at a time when they have limited access to rescue the airway, particularly when the patient is under the surgical drapes. Nonetheless, the LMA remains an extremely useful airway device that facilitates superb ventilation during surgery and allows rapid recovery with minimal coughing and straining in many patients.

Maintenance

The decision to allow children to breathe spontaneously or to artificially ventilate then depends on how the airway has been secured, the type and duration of surgery, and the depth of anaesthesia required. If the airway is likely to be difficult or the procedure is long, it is wise to secure the airway with an endotracheal tube and to ventilate to normocapnia using a non-depolarising muscle relaxant. Anaesthesia can be maintained either using total intravenous anaesthesia (TIVA) with propofol or with an inhalational technique, using a volatile agent such as sevoflurane, desflurane or isoflurane with or without nitrous oxide. TIVA with propofol is associated with less PONV, especially in children undergoing strabismus surgery.[29,30]

Anaesthesia for Specific Ophthalmic Surgery

Examination under Anaesthesia

Children may require direct fundoscopy, refraction, evaluation of tumours, IOP measurements, visual evoked responses, or electroretinography. Cooperation at such an early age is difficult or even impossible and these procedures may have to be performed under a general anaesthetic to insure complete immobility of the head. Anaesthesia may have to be repeated and the duration of procedures may vary. The children may be admitted as day cases, and clear instructions regarding preoperative fasting must be given to the parents. These procedures may be safely performed with the airway maintained by a laryngeal mask airway. As the oculo-cardiac reflex can occur, IV access and full monitoring must be used throughout.

Lacrimal Surgery

Children may present with an obstructed naso-lacrimal duct. The patency of the duct is checked under anaesthesia with the passage of a lacrimal probe through the puncta. Sterile saline or fluorescein may be injected and these may appear in, and contaminate, the naso-pharyngeal airway. Sometimes a silicone tube may be inserted for stenting, whilst some patients may require later dacryocystorhinostomy. The procedure is usually short and is managed as a day case. If large volumes of saline or fluorescein are to be used during the procedure, protection of the airway by endotracheal tube and throat pack may be required. If the surgeon confirms that little or no irrigation will take place, a laryngeal mask airway may be appropriate. In any case preparations for frequent naso-pharyngeal suctioning should be done. Full monitoring must be used throughout.

Anaesthesia for paediatric dacrocystorrhinostomy requires general anaesthesia with endotracheal intubation and packing of the pharynx to prevent contamination of the larynx with blood. The surgery may involve soft tissue and bone and is surgically stimulating.

Retinopathy of Prematurity (ROP)

Retinopathy of prematurity occurs in children who have usually received above atmospheric concentrations of oxygen in their earlier life.[31] Occasional reports describe premature infants who did not receive oxygen but nonetheless developed retinopathy.[32] The disease has been reported in infants of normal birth weight, in infants with cyanotic heart disease and in those delivered prematurely because of placental abruption following intrauterine bleeding.[33,34]

ROP is an abnormal proliferation of vascular tissue in the retina.[35] Normal retinal development involves the outward migration of mesenchyme from the optic disc. The nasal edge is closer and matures earlier during gestation. The temporal retina does not reach full maturation until 44 weeks after conception, and it is in this region that ROP most frequently occurs. Normally as the mesenchyme advances it differentiates into a fine capillary network.[35] In ROP, proliferation of undifferentiated primitive mesenchymal cells occurs forming arteriovenous shunts. Spontaneous regression of the disease with differentiation of shunt cells to capillaries occurs in 85% of cases. However, growth of these cells past the internal limiting membrane of the retina into vitreous body, leads to traction, retinal detachment and blindness.[35] Originally this condition was linked with uncontrolled oxygen usage, and the incidence fell in term infants with more controlled oxygen usage. The relationship between oxygen and ROP is more complex than originally thought, as some infants developed ROP despite never having received supplemental oxygen.

Today, ROP is predominately a disease of very low birth weight infants, especially those born below 1000 g birth weight.[36] The diagnosis is made clinically by indirect ophthalmoscopy, after prior pupillary dilatation. The condition is staged as follows:[37]

Stage 1   Demarcation Line — A thin white line of demarcation in the periphery of the retina separating the vascular retina anteriorly from the vascularised retina posteriorly.

Stage 2   Ridge — The line is more extensive and forms a ridge.

Stage 3   Proliferation — Vascular proliferation immediately posterior to the ridge.

Stage 4   Retinal detachment (subtotal.)

Stage 5   Retinal detachment (total.)

Plus (+) is added if the following signs of activity are seen:

- Tortuosity and engorgement of retinal vessels;
- vascular engorgement of retinal vessels;
- vitreous haze;
- pupil rigidity.

The following screening programme is advocated:[38,39]

- All infants less than 1500 g birth weight or less than 13 weeks gestational age;
- the first examination should be 6–7 weeks after birth;
- examination should be undertaken every 2 weeks;
- if stage 1 or 2 disease is present regular examination is necessary until the process of resolution is under way;
- signs of plus disease are ominous.

The treatment of ROP is directed toward preventing further proliferation of the retinal vascular tissue.[40,41] It is the tethering and contraction of this leash of vessels that leads to retinal detachment and blindness. The goals of surgery are to stop progression and to repair any existing retinal defects. Cryotherapy, which destroys the abnormal retina vasculature, saves vision in infants with severe disease, and therapy needs to be started within days of recognition of threshold disease.[42] Buckling of the sclera may be required if there is a posterior retinal detachment, whilst more rarely vitrectomy may also be required. Air or sulphur hexafluoride may be injected into the posterior chamber in an attempt to facilitate the repair of a detached retina. Ideally nitrous oxide should not be used (see Chapter 12). Nitrous oxide rapidly diffuses into the gas bubble and this may cause a rapid rise in IOP sufficient to occlude the blood supply to the retina. Rapid diffusion of nitrous oxide out of the bubble after discontinuing it in the inspired gas mixture may also have detrimental effects.

Anaesthesia for this procedure presents multiple problems in this patient group. They are often still premature, with all the complications of a long SCBU stay. They often have bronchopulmonary dysplasia and are still oxygen dependent, in addition to all the problems of anaesthetising a well neonate. The procedure often takes more than an hour; therefore the procedure must be performed in a hospital with the facilities to anaesthetise and manage neonates pre- and post operatively. Extubation may prove to be difficult in these premature babies and the facility for prolonged ventilation must be available because postoperative ventilation is often necessary. Regional anaesthesia is not suitable for this patient group. The use of a LMA is also inappropriate. Endotracheal intubation with neuromuscular blockade and intermittent positive pressure ventilation is indicated. Often inhalational induction is performed, as vascular access may be difficult. Once the child is asleep a vein may be cannulated and neuromuscular relaxant administered. Intravenous therapy will be necessary, and close control of serum glucose may require IV dextrose and saline administration. The use of forced air warming systems, of raised room temperatures, and of overhead heaters may be necessary to maintain normothermia, which is most important.

Caffeine 10 mg kg^{-1} may be used to reduce the incidence of postoperative apnoea.

Strabismus Surgery

Strabismus correction represents the commonest ophthalmic operation undertaken on children. Strabismus is a deviation of one eye relative to the visual axis of the other eye. It may occur in any plane or direction. Surgery involves a repositioning of the extraocular muscles either by strengthening (resection) or weakening (recession). Adjustable suture surgery allows the surgeon to adjust the alignment of the eye after the end of operation and requires a patient who is awake and cooperative, without muscle relaxation. Sometimes a brief anaesthetic is required to adjust the suture.

For children aged under four years, the majority of anaesthetists use neuromuscular blocking agents to facilitate endotracheal intubation,[43] with increasing use of the laryngeal mask airway with increasing age.

Specific problems posed by strabismus surgery in children include:

- Overall anaesthetic technique;
- paralysis and controlled ventilation versus spontaneously breathing;
- endotracheal intubation versus use of the laryngeal mask airway;
- postoperative pain relief;
- postoperative nausea and vomiting;
- the oculo-cardiac reflex;
- the risk of malignant hyperpyrexia.

Although separate, in many respects these problems are interconnected.

Strabismus surgery has been not considered particularly painful surgery. It is usually undertaken as a day case, with few good studies looking at the requirements and effectiveness of analgesia in the home environment. In hospital, many anaesthetists would avoid the use of opioids. Intraoperative topical local anaesthesia is used by many. The addition of topical ketorolac 0.5% ophthalmic solution, in addition to paracetamol, does not improve postoperative analgesia.[44]

Postoperative nausea and vomiting remains a major problem following strabismus correction. Historically, rates above 40% have frequently been published, which may be due to a wide range of patient, surgical and anaesthetic factors.[45] All elements must be considered together rather than isolation of a single factor if low vomiting rates are to occur. A large number of studies have looked at the use of individual drugs at varying doses against the background of different anaesthetic techniques.[45] Varying degrees of success are reported.

Over the last five years, a range of studies have looked at a number of antiemetics including ondansetron, metoclopramide and droperidol, singly and in combination, before and after operations.[46–51] The standardised anaesthetic technique has often been endotracheal intubation with controlled ventilation. The results are very similar. All quote statistical improvement over placebo but the 24-hour emesis rate remains at a disappointing 25–30%. In a single study (with small numbers), Clonidine 4 µg kg^{-1}

orally approximately 100 minutes before a standardised propofol infusion, nitrous oxide technique, produced complete lack of emesis in the first 24 hours in 93% of children after a strabismus surgery (as against 67% with benzodiazepine pre-med).[52]

Allen et al.[53] have proposed that stimulation of a trigemino-vagal reflex arc may explain the high vomiting rate with this type of surgery. The oculo-cardiac reflex shares the same neuronal pathway, with the bradycardia being the only objective feature of the vaso-vagal response in an anaesthetised patient. In a study of 79 children (defining the oculo-cardiac reflex as a fall in heart rate of greater than 10% or an arrhythmia), they found a statistically significant association between the oculo-cardiac reflex and postoperative vomiting. They went on to propose blockade of the afferent limb of this reflex arc by regional analgesia as a potential method of reducing nausea and vomiting.[53]

Strabismus Surgery and Malignant Hyperthermia

It has been assumed that anaesthesia for strabismus correction is associated with a higher occurrence rate for malignant hyperpyrexia than other operative groups. This was based on two factors:

- There is a far higher incidence of masseter spasm following suxamethonium in children for strabismus surgery than other operations (2.8% vs 0.72%).
- Strabismus is considered by some to represent an underlying myopathy.

The definition of what constitutes masseter spasm and its relationship to the development of malignant hyperpyrexia has been documented.[54] Similarly the relationship between the muscular dystrophies (in particular Duchenne Muscular Dystrophy) and malignant hyperpyrexia is also not straightforward.[55] The only muscular dystrophy clearly associated with malignant hyperpyrexia is a very rare dystrophy, Central Core Disease. Its presentation is variable from neonatal hypotonia, delay in reaching motor milestones in infancy, to a mild non-progressive motor weakness often not being diagnosed until later life. Its name is derived from the histological appearance of degenerated regions in the muscle cell. It shares with malignant hyperpyrexia an autosomal-dominant inheritance and some families have co-segregation of the two conditions on a small region of chromosome 19.[56]

Ten years ago, the Malignant Hyperpyrexia Registry in the United States received a series of reports of cardiac arrests on induction of anaesthesia involving suxamethonium in apparently healthy children. Almost all these cases occurred in male children under eight years of age. Subsequently investigation identified that many of these children were subsequently found to have a previously unrecognised muscular dystrophy with suxamethonium precipitating hyperkalaemia, and a life-threatening arrhythmia.[57] Since it is difficult to identify which patients are at risk, suxamethonium should be reserved for emergency intubation or in instances when immediate securing of the airway is necessary.

The oculo-cardiac reflex may occur in these patients and appropriate measures should be taken (see Chapter 3). This reflex can be prevented by the topical application of local anaesthetic solution to the muscle after opening the conjunctiva, peribulbar block, or a single medial periconal injection.[58]

Congenital Cataract Surgery

A cataract distorts image formation by interfering with the passage of light through the lens to the retina. Visual development in early infancy depends on retinal stimulation. This retinal activity must occur before two years of age or sooner because blindness is irretrievable beyond this time. It is therefore essential to perform cataract excision surgery as soon as possible following the diagnosis of a congenital cataract.[59–62]

The diagnosis of a congenital cataract carries the implication of other associated medical conditions (see Table 1). Many are idiopathic, but they may be associated with several, anaesthetically important, syndromes. Congenital cataract can occur in children born to mothers suffering from any of a number of infections, including rubella during the first trimester of pregnancy, toxoplasmosis, cytomegalovirus, or herpes simplex. Certain inherited conditions, including metabolic disorders, such as galactosemia, or chromosomal disorders, such as trisomy 21, have a high incidence of cataract. In Marfan's syndrome the lens can be subluxated (ectopia lentis) at birth, and this later becomes cloudy, requiring extraction.

The basic principle of the surgical procedure is to aspirate lens material by phacoemulsification through an incision near the limbus. Pupillary dilation with mydriatics is often necessary although some surgeons prefer to infuse epinephrine (1:200,000) continuously through a needle in the anterior chamber.[63] There is a potential risk of epinephrine being absorbed and this may lead to intense vasoconstriction and systemic absorption, but generally no ill effects have been observed. This may be due to a higher threshold for dysrhythmias in children after epinephrine.[64]

Glaucoma

If the outflow of aqueous humour is obstructed for whatever reasons, the IOP will increase leading to glaucoma. It can occur as a developmental problem, following cataract surgery, or ocular trauma. Many diseases such as von Recklinghausen syndrome, Sturge-Weber syndrome, and craniofacial malformations are associated with glaucoma. Repeated anaesthetics may be required for examination and diagnosis. Surgery may involve goniotomy or trabeculectomy to create an exit for aqueous

Table 1. Medical conditions which may be present in patients with congenital cataract.

Metabolic disorders	Chromosomal disorders	Infections
Galactosemia	Down's syndrome	TORCH infections
Diabetes mellitus	Trisomy 18	Varicella-zoster
Hypocalcaemia		
Lowe syndrome		
Alport syndrome		

humour. Cryotherapy is sometimes required to destroy the ciliary body and decrease aqueous production.

General anaesthesia, either using a laryngeal mask airway with spontaneous ventilation or an endotracheal tube and controlled ventilation, is satisfactory.[42] However, anaesthetic considerations must include awareness of associated medical problems, and the technique is modified accordingly.

Tumour Surgery

Children may present with either benign (capillary haemangioma, lymphangioma) or malignant tumours (rhabdomyosarcoma, retinoblastoma). Retinoblastoma is the most common eye tumour in children and is diagnosed and treated during the first three years of life. This may involve cryotherapy, photocoagulation, enucleation, chemotherapy or radiation (see Chapter 13).

Repeated anaesthetics are required. Anaesthesia for radiotherapy is short but may be repeated within days or weeks. During radiation therapy, the anaesthetist and monitoring may be some distance from the child. Full monitoring and control of the airway is mandatory. Anaesthesia for enucleation is more hazardous and the oculo-cardiac reflex frequently occurs (see Chapters 3 and 13).

Perforating Eye Injury

Eye trauma commonly occurs in children. The eye must be examined, and if there is a wound, it must be explored to remove any foreign body and/or to repair the injury. The principles and approach to anaesthesia for perforating eye injury is similar to adults. It is important to avoid any activity during induction that may increase IOP such as coughing, crying, an uncontrollable urge to rub the eye, and vomiting. Gastric emptying cannot be assumed to be complete and the use of sedatives and opiates may increase the risk of aspiration and vomiting. The use of antiemetics (metoclopramide may enhance gastric emptying) and H_2 blockers may be beneficial.

Postoperative Management

Routine Extubation

Opinions vary as to when the child should be extubated after surgery. Removal of an LMA is usually smooth, but if an endotracheal tube has been used to secure the airway, its removal can be associated with coughing, which may lead to an increased IOP. Coughing may also increase the tendency to bleed from the wound or into the eye if haemostasis is poor or impractical. Some anaesthetists use lidocaine spray or gel before intubation, whilst others may decide to extubate the child at the deeper plane of anaesthesia. Local anaesthesia to the airway delays the time for the child to restart oral intake, and is of poorly proven benefit.

Monitoring

Monitoring should be continued in the postoperative recovery room. Children are prone to develop hypoxia more quickly than adults, so supplemental oxygen should be administered during transfer and until the child is awake.

Postoperative Nausea and Vomiting (PONV)

Ophthalmological surgery is associated with a varying incidence of PONV and is most common after strabismus surgery in children where the incidence ranges from 40–88%.[64–66] It can occur in both early and late postoperative phases and continue for 24 hours. Various theories have been put forward to explain the high incidence of vomiting including the oculo-emetic reflex, postoperative distortion of vision, response to early fluid intake following day-case surgery, or motion sickness.[67] Whatever the reasons, antiemetics may only slightly reduce the incidence. An anaesthetic technique that avoids the use of intraoperative and postoperative opiates, inhalational agents and nitrous oxide may reduce the incidence. One of the lowest incidences of PONV has been reported following TIVA with propofol, even if supplemented by low dose fentanyl, sufentanil or nitrous oxide.[29,30,68] Prophylactic use of various antiemetics such as ondansetron,[69] granisetron,[70] low-dose droperidol,[71–73] metoclopramide,[74] or phenothiazines has reduced the incidence but has not completely abolished it. Hyoscine transdermal patch,[75] acupuncture and acupressure appear to have a marginal benefit.[76,77] A highly successful regimen is ondansetron 50 µg kg^{-1} combined with dexamethasone 150 µg kg^{-1} given intravenously just prior to the conclusion of surgery.[78–80] Dexamethasone is especially useful because of its prolonged duration of action and its ability to improve analgesia as well. The highest risk of PONV is in those who are female, are younger in age, and have a history of PONV and/or motion sickness, despite utmost care.[67]

Pain Control

Assessment of pain in children is difficult, but ophthalmic procedures in children are not usually associated with as much pain as other procedures. Restlessness in the recovery area may be due to factors other than pain, such as thirst, hunger, disorientation, strange environment, and absence of parents. Where there is an expectation of postoperative pain, local anaesthetic block techniques may be used, but their use may increase the incidence of complications. Topical local anaesthetic drops during strabismus surgery are effective postoperatively, but the onset of pain once the local anaesthetic has worn off can be distressing and may require opiate analgesia to achieve control. Opiates alone may be used to provide pain relief but are associated with an increased incidence of PONV. The administration of an NSAID rectally after induction of anaesthesia is usually helpful, if not contraindicated. Rectal acetaminophen is very useful, but must be given in adequate doses after induction of anaesthesia and prior to surgery. A dose of 40 mg kg^{-1} is recommended. Following this dose, parents must be warned not to give additional acetaminophen for at least six hours. Once the child is awake, oral therapy is effective. This is best accomplished by instructing parents to give an NSAID, followed two hours later by acetaminophen, followed two hours later by the NSAID, and so forth, so that the child is able to have something for pain every two hours if necessary. After 24–36 hours postoperatively, acetaminophen alone is usefully sufficient.

References

1   Ausinch B, Graves SA, Munson ES, Levy NS. Intraocular pressures in children during isoflurane and halothane anesthesia. *Anesthesiology.* 1975; 42:167–172.
2   Joshi C, Bruce DL. Thiopental and succinylcholine: Action on intraocular pressure. *Anesth Analg.* 1975; 54:471–475.
3   Thomson MF, Brock-Utne JG, Bean P, Welsh N, Downing JW. Anaesthesia and intraocular pressure: a comparative of total intravenous anaesthesia using etomidate with conventional inhalation anaesthesia. *Anaesthesia.* 1982; 37:758–761.
4   Mirakhur RK, Shepherd WF, Darrah WC. Propofol or thiopentone: Effects on intraocular pressure associated with induction of anaesthesia and tracheal intubation (facilitated with suxamethonium). *Br J Anaesth.* 1987; 59:431–436.
5   Leopald IH, Comroe JH Jr. Effect of intramuscular administration of morphine, atropine, scopolamine on the human eye. *Arch Ophthalmol.* 1948; 40:285–290.
6   Mostafa SM, Lockhart A, Kumar D, Bayoumi M. Comparison of effects of fentanyl and alfentanil on intra-ocular pressure. A double-blind controlled trial. *Anaesthesia.* 1986; 41:493–498.
7   Yoshikawa K, Murai Y. The effect of ketamine on intraocular pressure in children. *Anesth Analg.* 1971; 50:199–202.
8   Zimmerman AA, Funk KJ, Tidwell JL. Propofol and alfentanil prevent the increase in intraocular pressure caused by succinylcholine and endotracheal intubation during a rapid sequence induction of anesthesia. *Anesth Analg.* 1996; 83:814–817.
9   Litwiller RW, DiFazio CA, Rushia EL. Pancuronium and intraocular pressure. *Anesthesiology.* 1975; 42:750–752.
10 Schneider MJ, Stirt JA, Finholt DA. Atracurium, vecuronium and intraocular pressure in humans. *Anesth Analg.* 1986; 65:877–882.
11 Murphy DF, Eustace P, Unwin A, Magner JB. Atracurium and intraocular pressure. *Br J Anaesth.* 1985; 69:673–675.
12 Maharaj RJ, Humphrey D, Kaplan N, Kadwa H, Blignaut P, Brock-Utne JG, Welsh N. Effects of atracurium on intraocular pressure. *Br J Anaesth.* 1984; 56:459–463
13 Polarz H, Bohrer H, von Tabouillot W, Martin E, Tetz M, Volcker HE. Comparative effects of atracurium and vecuronium on intraocular pressure. *Ger J Ophthalmol.* 1995; 4:91–93.
14 Pandey K, Badola RP, Kumar S, Time course of intraocular hypertension produced by suxamethonium. *Br J Anaesth.* 1972; 44:191–196.
15 Metz HS, Venkatesh B. Succinylcholine and intraocular pressure. *J Pediatr Ophthalmol Strabismus.* 1981; 18:12–14.
16 Berler DK, The oculocardiac reflex. *Am J Ophthalmol.* 1963; 56:954–959.
17 Alexander JP. Reflex disturbances of cardiac rhythm during ophthalmic surgery. *Br J Ophthalmol.* 1975; 59:518–524.
18 Meyers EF, Tomeldan SA. Glycopyrrolate compared with atropine in prevention of the oculocardiac reflex during eye-muscle surgery. *Anesthesiology.* 1979; 51:350–352.
19 Morselli PL. Clinical pharmacokinetics in neonates. In: Gibaldi M, Prescott L, editors. Handbook of clinical pharmacokinetics. Adis Health Science Press, New York, 1983. p 79.

20   Katoh T, Ikeda K. Minimum alveolar concentration of sevoflurane in children. *Br J Anaesth.* 1992; 68:139–141.

21   Olsson GL, Hallen B, Hambraeus-Jonzon K. Aspiration during anaesthesia: a computer-aided study of 185,358 anaesthetics. *Acta Anaesthesiol Scand.* 1986; 30:84–92.

22   Vassalo SA, Ferrari LR. A practice of anesthesia for infants and children. In: Cote, Todres, Ryan, Goudsouzian, 3rd Edition 2001, Philadelphia, PA, USA: WB Saunders Company, 479–492.

23   Cote CJ. Preoperative fasting: is the answer clear? *J Pediatr.* 1998; 132:1077–1078.

24   Meakin G, Dingwall AE, Addison GM. Effects of fasting and oral premedication on the pH and volume of gastric aspirate in children. *Br J Anaesth.* 1987; 59:678–682.

25   Splinter WM, Stewart JA, Muir JG. Large volumes of apple juice preoperatively do not affect gastric pH and volume in children. *Can J Anaesth.* 1990; 37:36–39.

26   Patel DK, Keeling PA, Newman GB, Radford P. Induction dose of propofol in children. *Anaesthesia.* 1988; 43:949–952.

27   Watcha MF, Simeon RM, White PF, Stevens JL. Effects of propofol on the incidence of postoperative vomiting after strabimus surgery in pedriatic outpatients. *Anesthiology.* 1991; 75:204–209.

28   Watcha MF, White PF, Tychsen L, et al. Comparative effects of laryngeal mask airway and endotracheal tube insertion on intraocular pressure in children. *Anesth Analg.* 1992; 75:355–360.

29   Snellen FT, Vanacker B, Van Aken H. Propofol-nitrous oxide versus thiopental sodium-isoflurane-nitrous oxide for strabismus surgery in children. *J Clin Anesth.* 1993; 5:37–41.

30   Tramer M, Moore A, McQuay H. Meta-analytic comparison of prophylactic antiemetic efficacy for postoperative nausea and vomiting: propofol anaesthesia vs omitting nitrous oxide vs total i.v. Anaesthesia with propofol. *Br J Anaesth.* 1997; 78:256–259.

31   Campbell K. Intensive oxygen therapy as a possible cause of retrolental fibroplasia A clinical approach. *Med J Aust.* 1951; 2:48–50.

32   Adamkin DH, Shott RJ, Cook LN, Andrews BF. Nonhyperoxic retrolental fibroplasia. *Pediatrics.* 1977; 60:828–830.

33   Brockhurst RJ, Chisti MI. Cicatricial retrolental fibroplasia: Its occurrence without oxygen administration and in full term infants. *Albrecht Von Graefes Arch Klin Exp Ophthalmol.* 1975; 195:113–128.

34   Kalina RE, Hodson WA, Morgan BC. Retrolental fibroplasia in a cynotic infant. *Pediatrics.* 1972; 50:765–768.

35   Flynn JT, Bancalari E, Bachynski BN, Buckley EB, Bawol R, Goldberg R, Cassady J, Schiffman J, Feuer, W, Gillings. Retinopathy of prematurity. Diagnosis, severity and natural history. *Ophthalmology.* 1987; 94:620–629.

36   Flynn JT. Acute proliferative retrolental fibroplasia: Multivariate risk analysis. *Trans Am Ophthalmol Soc.* 1983; 81:549–591.

37   The International Committee for the Classification of the Late Stages of Retinopathy of Prematurity. An international classification of retinopathy of prematurity II. The classification of retinal detachment. *Arch Ophthalmol.* 1987; 105:906–912.

38   American Academy of Pediatrics Committee on Practice and Ambulatory Medicine. Section on Ophthalmology: Eye examination and vision screening in infants, children, and young adults. *Pediatrics.* 1996; 98:153–157.

39   American Academy of Pediatrics, the American Association for Pediatric Ophthalmology and Strabismus, and the American Academy of Ophthalmology. Screening examination of premature infants for retinopathy of prematurity: A Joint Statement. *Pediatrics.* 1997; 100:273.

40   Hirose T, Lou PL. Retinopathy of prematurity. *Int Ophthalmol Clin.* 1986; 26:1–23.

41   Flynn JT. Oxygen and retrolental fibroplasias: update and challenge. *Anesthesiology.* 1984; 60:397–399.

42   Cryotherapy for Retinopathy of Prematurity Cooperative Group. Multicenter trial of cryotherapy for retinopathy of prematurity. Preliminary results. *Arch Ophthalmol.* 1988; 106:471–479.

43   Dell R, Williams B. Anaesthesia for strabismus surgery: a regional survey. *Br J Anaesth.* 1999; 82:5:761–763.

44   Bridge HS, Montgomery CJ, Kennedy RA, Merrick PM. Analgesic efficacy of ketorolac 0.5% ophthalmic solution (Accular) in paediatric strabismus surgery. *Paediatr Anaesth.* 2000; 10:521–526.

45   Tramer M, Moore A, McQuay H. Prevention of vomiting after paediatric strabismus surgery: a systematic review using the numbers-needed-to-treat method. *Br J Anaesth.* 1995; 75:556–561.

46   Scuderi PE, Weaver RG Jr, James RL, Mims G, Elliott WG, Weeks DB. A randomized, double-blind, placebo controlled comparison of droperidol, ondansetron, and metoclopramide for the prevention of vomiting following outpatient strabismus surgery in children. *J Clin Anesth.* 1997; 9:551–558.

47   Welters ID, Menges T, Graf M, Beikirch C, Menzebach A, Hempelmann G. Reduction of postoperative nausea and vomiting by dimenhydrinate suppositories after strabismus surgery in children. *Anesth Analg.* 2000; 90:311–314.

48   Sadhasivam S, Shende D, Madan R. Prophylactic ondansetron in prevention of postoperative nausea and vomiting following pediatric strabismus surgery: a dose-response study. *Anesthesiology.* 2000; 92:1035–1042.

49   Saiah M, Borgeat A, Ruetsch YA, Seifert B, Klainguti G. Myopexy (Faden) results in more postoperative vomiting after strabismus surgery in children. *Acta Anaesthesiol Scand.* 2001; 45:59–64.

50   Bowhay AR, May HA, Rudnicka AR, Booker PD. A randomized controlled trial of the antiemetic effect of three doses of ondansetron after strabismus surgery in children. *Paediatr Anaesth.* 2001; 11:215–221.

51   Rusch D, Happe W, Wulf H. [Postoperative nausea and vomiting following stabismus surgery in children. Inhalation anesthesia with sevoflurane-nitrous oxide in comparison with intravenous anesthesia with propofol-remifentanil. *Anaesthesist.* 1999; 48(2):80–88.

52   Handa F, Fujii Y. The efficacy of oral clonidine premedication in the prevention of postoperative vomiting in children following strabismus surgery. *Paediatr Anaesth.* 2001; 11:71–74.

53   Allen LE, Sudesh S, Sandramouli S, Cooper G, McFarlane D, Willshaw HE. The association between the oculocardiac reflex and post-operative vomiting in children undergoing strabismus surgery. *Eye.* 1998; 12:193–196.

54   Rosenberg H, Shutack JG. Variants of malignant hyperthermia. Special problems for the paediatric anaesthesiologist. *Paediatr Anaesth.* 1996; 6:87–93.

55   Morris P. Duchenne muscular dystrophy: a challenge for the anaesthetist. *Paediatr Anaesth.* 1997; 7:1–4.

56   Curran JL, Hall WJ, Halsall PJ, Hopkins PM, Iles DE, Markham AF, McCall SH, Robinson RL, West SP, Bridges LR, Ellis FR. Segregation of malignant hyperthermia, central core disease and chromosome 19 markers. *Br J Anaesth.* 1999; 83:217–222.

57   Larach MG, Rosenberg H, Gronert GA, Allen GC. Hyperkalemic cardiac arrest during anesthesia in infants and children with occult myopathies. *Clin Pediatr (Phila).* 1997; 36:9–16.

58   Fry RA. Postoperative pain and vomiting may be decreased by regional local anesthetic block. *Reg Anesth Pain Med.* 1999; 24:582–583.

59   Brett CM, Zwass MS, France NK. Pediatric Anesthesia. In: Gregory GA, editor. Churchill Livingstone, New York, 1994. p 685.

60   Calhoun JH. Cataracts in children. *Pediatr Clin North Am.* 1983; 30:1061–1069.

61   Enoch JM, Campos EC. Helping the aphakic neonate to see. *Int Ophthalmol.* 1985; 8:237–248.

62   Lambert SR, Drack AV. Infantile cataracts. *Surv Ophthalmol.* 1996; 40:427–458.

63   Smith RB, Douglas H, Petruscak J, Breslin P. Safety of intraocular adrenaline with halothane anaesthesia. *Br J Anaesth.* 1972; 44:1314–1317.

64   Hardy JF, Charest J, Girouard G, Lepage Y. Nausea and vomiting after strabismus surgery in preschool children. *Can Anaesth Soc J.* 1986; 33:57–62.

65   Cohen MM, Cameron CB, Duncan PG. Pediatric anesthesia morbidity and mortality in the perioperative period. *Anesth Analg.* 1990; 70:160–167.

66   Karlsson E, Larsson LE, Nilsson K. Postanaesthetic nausea in children. *Acta Anaesthesiol Scand.* 1990; 34:515–518.

67   Lerman J. Surgical and patient factors involved in postoperative nausea and vomiting. *Br J Anaesth.* 1992; 69:24S-32S.

68   Wilhelm S, Standl T. Does propofol have advantages over isoflurane for sufentanil supplemented anesthesia in children for strabismus surgery? *Anasthesiol Intensivmed Notfallmed Schmerzther.* 1996; 31:414–419.

69   Davis A, Krige S, Moyes D. A double-blind randomized prospective study comparing ondansetron with droperidol in the prevention of emesis following strabismus surgery. *Anaesth Intensive Care.* 1995; 23:438–443.

70   Fujii Y, Saitoh Y, Tanaka H, Toyooka H. Combination of granisetron and droperidol for the prevention of vomiting after paediatric strabismus surgery. *Paediatr Anaesth.* 1999; 9:329–333.

71   Abramowitz MD, Oh TH, Epstein BS, Ruttimann UE, Friendly DS. The antiemetic effect of droperidol following outpatient strabismus surgery in children. *Anesthesiology.* 1983; 59:579–583.

72   Lerman J, Eustis S, Smith DR. Effect of droperidol pretreatment on postanesthetic vomiting in children undergoing strabismus surgery. *Anesthesiology.* 1986; 65:322–325.

73   Brown RE Jr, James DJ, Weaver RG, Wilhoit RD, Bauman LA. Low-dose droperidol versus standard-dose droperidol for prevention of postoperative vomiting after pediatric strabismus surgery. *J Clin Anesth.* 1991; 3:306–309.

74   Broadman LM, Ceruzzi W, Patane PS, Hannallah RS, Ruttimann U, Friendly D. Metoclopramide reduces the incidence of vomiting following strabismus surgery in children. *Anesthesiology.* 1990; 72:245–248.

75   Horimoto Y, Tomie H, Hanzawa K, Nishida Y. Scopolamine patch reduces postoperative emesis in paediatric patients following strabismus surgery. *Can J Anaesth.* 1991; 38:441–444.

76   Schlager A, Boehler M, Puhringer F. Korean hand acupressure reduces postoperative vomiting in children after strabismus surgery. *Br J Anaesth.* 2000; 85:267–270.

77   Schlager A, Offer T, Baldissera I. Laser stimulation of acupuncture point P6 reduces postoperative vomiting in children undergoing strabismus surgery. *Br J Anaesth.* 1998; 81:529–532.

78   Busoni P, Crescioli M, Agostino R, Sestini G. Vomiting and common paediatric surgery. *Paediatr Anaesth.* 2000; 10:639–643.

79   Fujii Y, Saitoh Y, Tanaka H, Toyooka H. Prophylactic therapy with combined granisetron and dexamethasone for the prevention of post-operative vomiting in children. *Eur J Anaesthesiol.* 1999; 16:376–379.

80   Fujii Y, Tanaka H, Toyooka H. Granistron and dexamethasone provide more improved
      prevention of postoperative emesis than granisetron alone in children. *Can J Anaesth.*
      1996; 43:1229–1232.

11

General Anaesthesia for Ophthalmic Surgery

Prof Chris Dodds

Aims and Objectives

This chapter will cover those aspects of anaesthetic care that relate to the decision to choose a general anaesthetic instead of a local anaesthetic for ophthalmic procedures. Key areas in this decision-making process are the assessment of the patient, the procedure and the operating team. These will be covered in turn, with the details of appropriate anaesthetic agents and techniques discussed where relevant. An understanding of the skills and attitudes necessary to provide safe general anaesthesia will be developed through this chapter.

Introduction and Context

The current drive for rapid turnover of patients for procedures such as cataract excision and lens implantation has biased the view of anaesthetists and surgeons with regard to the provision of services for ophthalmic surgery. The general anaesthetic techniques[1] that were in place before the explosion of peribulbar and now sub-Tenon's techniques are now largely historical (albeit safe and effective), yet they remain the comparative alternative in the minds of many practitioners when choices are being offered to patients or institutions. Recovery times from local anaesthetic blockade to being 'home ready' is indeed short (unless there are complications), yet general anaesthesia can now match this in skilled hands.[2] General anaesthesia avoids some of the complications associated with local anaesthesia; it is the only technique that has not resulted in a globe perforation.[3,4] Whilst local anaesthesia for cataract surgery is more widely practiced in the USA compared to Europe, postoperative untoward events with their associated poor visual outcome were almost four times more common in the USA[5] — perhaps the anaesthetic technique is important after all.

There is no ideal anaesthetic technique for any operation, local or general. This leads to the need to make an informed decision on which technique is most appropriate. Having a stand-alone centre where facilities for the safe administration of a general anaesthetic are lacking or where the skills of the anaesthetic personnel are focused in only one technique may bias this. Certainly in Europe the majority of ophthalmic surgical units are some distance from an acute hospital site and lack intensive care or even high dependency care facilities.

The requirements for an ideal anaesthetic technique are the subject of many anaesthetic examinations, and usually include goals such as:

- Pain-free surgery;
- rapid onset of anaesthesia;
- cardiovascular and respiratory stability;
- rapid recovery postoperatively;
- immobile operating field;
- reduced or normal intraocular pressure;
- no postoperative nausea and vomiting;
- no complications or drug toxicity;
- minimal metabolism of the active drug;
- no accumulation of metabolites.

However, these remain only a wish list and bear little relationship to the real world. What is needed is a series of agents that allow the necessary requirements for a successful procedure to be tailored to the condition of the patient who needs the operation. The majority of patients dealt with are either the very young or the elderly; there appears little demand from the fit and healthy.

Patient Factors

The ultimate indication for a general anaesthetic (see Table 1) may be the wish of the patient, but there are other indications that may carry as much weight. In practice children are more safely and humanely operated on under general anaesthesia. Elderly patients should be assessed to ascertain their ability to understand instructions and to cooperate. Many elderly patients are very deaf as well as having visual impairment and this is very debilitating. The deafness is often denied, being blamed on softly spoken carers or 'wax.' The patient's primary language may differ from that of the host country, and the stress of an operating procedure may erode his/her ability to maintain understanding of instructions. All of these may make a local technique more risky and should move the decision towards a general anaesthetic.

Medical conditions that can cause problems include the tremor of Parkinson's disease, which gets worse on attention and may lead to extreme head movement even if it is only affecting the limbs. Cognitive dysfunction may be subtle and well masked or there may be frank dementia. The disorientation caused by a day-care hospital admission can prove disabling for the patient. The ability of the patient to lie recum-

Table 1. Patient factors indicating the need for general anaesthesia.

• Children/neonates
• Inability to communicate
• Involuntary movement disorders
• Dementing disorders
• Deafness
• Severe respiratory failure
• Irritable coughing
• Orthopnoea
• Extreme anxiety
• Allergy to local anaesthetic agents
• Severe learning disability
• Hypersomnolence

bent for a reasonable period of time is vital, even for experienced phacoemulsification surgeons. Orthopnoea, severe respiratory failure or paroxysms of coughing all indicate the need to consider a general anaesthetic technique. The rare patient who is truly allergic to local anaesthetic agents is an obvious candidate.

Procedure-based Factors

Paediatric procedures are usually best performed under general anaesthesia and were discussed in more detail in the chapter on paediatric ophthalmic anaesthesia (see Chapter 10).

Adult surgery is dominated by the elderly and by the demand for correction of the visual impairment of cataracts and the field loss of glaucoma. The speed of cataract surgery in experienced hands belies the skill necessary to achieve a safe result, and the anaesthetic technique plays a major part in this process. However, whilst cataract and glaucoma surgery are the commonest procedures performed in ophthalmic practice, there are many other procedures that are of longer duration and may involve more intense stimulation of the operating site. These include vitroretinal surgery, adult strabismus surgery, corneal grafting and oculoplastic procedures.

Proprioceptive reflexes limit the time that immobility can be tolerated, and there are few patients who can lie still for more than 40 minutes without increasing discomfort. After an hour this discomfort will become more marked. For procedures that last longer than an hour the indications for a pure local anaesthetic technique are very limited. Techniques (see Chapter 8) for providing safe sedation during prolonged operations inevitably have an element of unpredictability in the depth of sedation, and may deepen to the level of true anaesthesia without the elementary safeguards inherent in general anaesthesia.

The procedures that determine anaesthetic technique involve the globe itself, the other contents of the orbit and the peri-orbital area including the lacrimal apparatus.

Globe-related Surgery

Complex vitreoretinal surgery is often prolonged and intermittently painful. It frequently involves indirect ophthalmoscopy in a darkened operating theatre, and may involve intravitreal injections of oils or inert gases, placing of compressive plombs around the globe, or cryotherapy. The operative requirements for this form of surgery are for a stable intraocular pressure, suppression of the oculocardiac, oculo-respiratory and oculo-emetic reflexes and a rapid pain-free return to consciousness.

Corneal surgery, especially where full-thickness grafting is planned, is rarely suitable for a local anaesthetic approach. This surgery is also more frequent in younger adults, who appear to be less stoical than their elders. Sudden changes in choroidal blood volume and in the episcleral venous pressure may severely compromise the operating field by marked swings in the intraocular pressure. These are commonly caused by coughing or hypertensive responses, which occur as often with a local technique as with a poorly conducted general anaesthetic.

Other procedures that involve the globe are the emergency treatment of a penetrating eye injury or the treatment of an evolving retinal detachment or haemorrhage following a needle injury from an attempted local block.

Orbital Procedures

Orbital procedures commonly involve the extraocular muscles or the eyelids. Infrequently conjunctival tumours such as lymphomas require extensive procedures and may lead to very painful eyes postoperatively. Strabismus surgery in the adult is more commonly associated with either trauma or undiagnosed muscle weakness. Increasingly both adult and paediatric operations for correction are being performed with an adjustable suture to allow precise balancing of the muscles and improved functional and cosmetic results. Return of normal muscle tone and visual fixation are important factors in the success of this operation and this may be delayed if there is residual motor or optic nerve blockade from local anaesthetic.

Extraorbital Surgery

The diseases of the lacrimal system become more prevalent with advancing age, and failure of drainage of tears is the most common reason for surgery outside the orbit. The traditional external approach[6] for dacryocystorhinostomy (DCR) has been partly replaced by laser DCR, which is much less likely to lead to blood loss than the traditional approach. It is a more rapid operation but does not appear to have such good long-term patency. Cosmetic procedures around the orbit are also becoming more common. These are often very painful postoperatively and may require opioid prescription as well as NSAIDs.

General Anaesthetic Techniques

The ideal general anaesthetic technique for ophthalmic surgery has to provide a pain-free and immobile eye for the surgeon with no alteration in intraocular pressure. This should be maintained as long as necessary and be followed by a rapid and complete recovery of the patient from the anaesthetic. The avoidance of coughing and straining on emergence from anaesthesia was of great importance historically when there were no fine suture materials and wounds were much larger and often were not water-tight. This is no longer the case, but coughing will still increase the IOP and should be limited if not completely avoided. The ocular reflexes to traction on, and compression of, the globe may lead to hypoxia and hypercarbia or bradycardia. Protection from the results of the vagal stimulation will require controlled ventilation in the majority of patients. Postoperative nausea and vomiting may be very troublesome and difficult to avoid with either local or general anaesthesia.

In these days of financial restraints, economy and cost-effectiveness are becoming more important aspects to consider within any anaesthetic context, and general anaesthesia for ophthalmic surgery is no exception.

The increased availability of continuous, real-time, monitoring of the patient and of improved anaesthetic machine performance has coincided with a greater use of very low-flow anaesthetic techniques. This has allowed anaesthetists to rely on direct observation of the patient rather than on a series of rote-learnt guidelines to deliver safe care. This has also led to a progressive reduction in the administered fresh gas flow rate, which has dramatically reduced the cost of volatile anaesthetic agent use[7] (where insoluble agents are used). Computerised intravenous pumps with sophisticated models for induction and maintenance of anaesthesia with intravenous agents are available and are proving cost effective. Finally, potent drugs that have a very short context-sensitive half-time are available to provide analgesia during prolonged and painful surgery.

Anaesthetists are now in the position to choose the anaesthetic in response to the patient's physical condition and deliver safe and satisfactory conditions for surgery. If the patient has severe pulmonary disease with unpredictable ventilation/perfusion gradients or frank shunting, gaseous anaesthesia can be avoided completely and a total intravenous technique can be used. If patients have severe renal or hepatic disease, volatile induction and maintenance of anaesthesia provides an effective alternative.[8]

Anaesthetic Drugs

There have been major advances in anaesthetic agents over the last few years. Many of these have been of great value to ophthalmic anaesthesia.

Volatile Anaesthetic Agents
The two new volatile anaesthetic agents — sevoflurane and desflurane — have transformed the ability to provide not only reliable general anaesthesia but also predictably

rapid and complete recovery from their effects. The duration of the procedure has very little impact on this recovery.

Sevoflurane is a methyl isopropyl ether and is both a noninflammable and a non-irritating volatile anaesthetic agent.

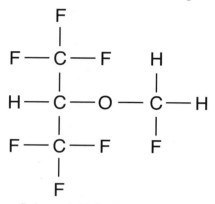

It has a MAC of 2% in young adults, a vapour pressure at 20° C of 160 mm Hg, and has a blood/brain solubility coefficient of 1.7 and a blood/gas solubility coefficient of 0.65. It is approximately 2–3% metabolised and has a MAC_{awake} of 0.6%. The nonirritant nature of sevoflurane has allowed its use as a gaseous induction agent as well as being useful for the maintenance of anaesthesia. The low solubilities indicate a potential for rapid variations in plasma concentration both for induction, for responding to changing surgical stimulation, and for recovery. The advantage of sevoflurane for ophthalmic surgery is the smooth induction and rapid recovery for operations lasting up to an hour. It can be used as a sole anaesthetic agent (Volatile Induction and Maintenance of Anaesthesia — VIMA) where high concentrations of 4–8% in oxygen are used for induction and then reduced for maintenance. The induction may be by either repeated high volume breaths or a single vital capacity inhalation followed by a voluntary breath hold. Once induction has been achieved, the inspired concentration is reduced to single MAC values and this is then continued for the duration of the surgery. Cardiovascular stability is well maintained and many patients who have had a VIMA technique would have one again (just as is the case with topical anaesthesia for instance).

The use of low fresh gas flow rates with sevoflurane, (especially if nitrous oxide is avoided obviating the need to wash out nitrogen) combined with its very low solubility makes it one of the cheapest volatile anaesthetic agents to use. It has little direct effect on intraocular pressure, although it will have an indirect effect if the patient is allowed to breathe spontaneously.

Sevoflurane does have a perceived problem in that it has several potentially harmful breakdown products. These include fluoride, and measured concentrations of fluoride can increase during surgery. They do not cause clinical problems at concentrations identified in humans. Compound A, an olefin that causes renal damage in rodents, is a breakdown product of sevoflurane that has been identified in closed circle systems. The production of both compound A and carbon monoxide can be avoided by using a lithium hydroxide based absorbent for carbon dioxide[9] or by maintaining humidification of the absorbent. It is one reason why the fresh gas flow rate in the USA is restricted to above 2 l min^{-1} although the rest of the world will reduce flows to 300 ml min^{-1}.

Desflurane has a MAC of 6% and a vapour pressure at 20° C of 664 mm Hg. It has a blood/brain solubility coefficient of 1.3, and a blood/gas solubility coefficient of 0.45. Only 0.02% of it can be recovered as metabolites, and it has a MAC$_{awake}$ of 0.6%.

It is much more irritant than sevoflurane to the airway and is less potent. Desflurane's pungency prevents its use for the induction of anaesthesia, but because plasma concentrations very quickly reach inhaled concentrations, it is an ideal agent for maintaining anaesthesia after an intravenous induction. It is not metabolised to any real extent and because of its very low solubility can be very rapidly titrated for maintenance and reversal of anaesthesia. It can cause sympathetic stimulation if the inhaled vapour concentration is raised too quickly, and the tachycardia and hypertensive response following this may cause problems in ophthalmic surgery. It is, like sevoflurane, very cost effective when used in a low flow system. Its prime advantage is in prolonged operations where the minimal absorption and metabolism make the time to move from MAC$_{asleep}$ to MAC$_{awake}$ almost independent of time administered.[10]

Other Anaesthetic Gases

Xenon is an inert noble gas that was identified to have anaesthetic properties over 50 years ago. It is the only inert gas that is anaesthetic below atmospheric pressure and it has a MAC of 71%. It is an effective analgesic in sub-anaesthetic concentrations, and is MAC additive. It is expensive, but increasingly available as a by-product from other gas manufacturing processes. It has been proposed as an alternative to nitrous oxide. It can only be given in closed systems and requires all of the in-built safety features in the anaesthetic machine necessary when administering a gas that can lead to a hypoxic gas mixture. It is more cardio-stable than nitrous oxide and less emetic, but it remains an uncertain agent in search of a role in general anaesthesia.

Nitrous oxide remains a very popular adjunct to the more potent volatile anaesthetic agents, but the problems associated with its use continue to question its place in modern anaesthesia.[11] It is believed to cause problems with the intravitreal gas used for tamponade in vitreoretinal surgery due to the differential diffusion characteristics of the two gases. It is highly emetic and in prolonged administration affects methionine synthetase activity.

Intravenous Agents

Propofol
The safety and effectiveness of propofol in maintaining or reducing intraocular pressure on induction and maintenance of anaesthesia has been well established. The cardiovascular effects of excessive dosage or speed of induction are well known and now usually avoided. It can be used as a total intravenous anaesthetic technique (TIVA) using computer or manually adjusted infusions or using a target-controlled model (Diprifusor^R for example).[12] The ability to adjust the effect site concentration and knowing the time to waking are tremendous advantages when dealing with frail elderly patients. One problem with the TIVA technique is a delayed recovery if the operation is prolonged. The accumulation of propofol due to the context-sensitive half-time means a delayed time to full recovery. In the majority of elective ophthalmic procedures this is rarely an issue. Propofol has an antiemetic action,[13] and this may be beneficial in ophthalmic procedures such as strabismus surgery where postoperative nausea and vomiting is common.

Remifentanil
This is the first opioid released into clinical practice that is metabolized by the plasma and tissue esterase system. Remifentanil is a potent opioid selective for μ-opioid receptors and it produces intense analgesia very rapidly. The μ-activity that it shares with other opioids causes respiratory depression, bradycardia, and severe skeletal muscle rigidity as well as the profound analgesia. The rigidity may be reduced or avoided if remifentanil is administered after induction of anaesthesia. It is such a potent respiratory depressant that the volume remaining in the priming volume of an intravenous cannula is enough to precipitate a respiratory arrest. However, the cardiovascular stability, marked analgesia and time-independent termination of action make it an ideal intraoperative opioid. The very predictable nature of remifentanil makes it ideal for ophthalmic surgery in ill or very frail patients. Remifentanil is most valuable in patients with severe chest disease where there is little or no place for prolonged respiratory depression after anaesthesia, and its predictable and complete metabolism ensure a return to the preoperative respiratory drive as soon as possible.

Neuromuscular Blocking Agents

The requirements of ophthalmic surgery for an immobile eye and maintained intraocular pressure usually indicates controlled ventilation, and, by inference, muscle relaxation. There is still a need for very rapidly acting drugs to achieve airway protection. Until recently, the depolarizing drug suxamethonium was the only safe agent, although it has problems with increasing intraocular pressure. Rocuronium, an ammonio-steroid, is fast acting in moderately high dosage and can achieve satisfactory intubating conditions within 60 seconds.[14]

There are several other recently released relaxant agents; of these, cisatracurium (one of the many isomers within atracurium) has advantages in still being metabolised by Hoffman elimination, and it has very little histamine release. This cardio-stability and reliable elimination make it very suitable for eye surgery in the elderly.

Longer-acting relaxants, such as doxacurium, have few indications within the scope of ophthalmic anaesthesia.

Other Anaesthetic Adjuncts

The prevention of the oculo-cardiac reflex is usually by the intravenous administration of anticholinergic drugs such as atropine. In the elderly this crosses the blood/brain barrier and can lead to confusion and cognitive dysfunction,[15] both of which are very problematic following eye surgery. Glycopyrrolate is a quaternary amine and does not cross into the brain. It causes less tachycardia and is longer acting. These considerations should limit the use of atropine to paediatric use or the management of acute and severe bradycardia. It should be avoided in the elderly.

Postoperative nausea and vomiting are very common after some ophthalmic procedures, such as strabismus surgery,[16] and frequently require active drug therapy. The more recent agents have not always proved to be of greater efficacy than the more established agents,[17,18] although propofol does reduce the incidence of nausea and vomiting compared to other induction agents. Combinations of ondansetron and dexamethasone have proved effective in children (see Chapter 10) but little has been documented in adult ophthalmic surgery.

Dilemmas with the Anaesthetic Technique

The combination of operations on the head with draping over the face and airway, darkened rooms and frail patients is a clear indication for protecting the airway during anaesthesia. The laryngeal mask airway has become one of the most frequently used airway devices and many practitioners also use it to artificially ventilate the patient. Endotracheal intubation remains the safest option, especially in children and the elderly. The advantages of the laryngeal mask airway (lower intraocular pressure after insertion,[19] fewer sore throats, minimal airway instrumentation) are balanced by the disadvantages of having no protection against aspiration and of very easy displacement by the surgical drapes especially if an armoured/flexible laryngeal mask airway is not used. Very large-scale studies into the safety or otherwise of ventilating through a laryngeal mask airway have been published. Although only a small number of patients are placed at risk in these studies, the complications are life threatening. For elective surgery, including the majority of ophthalmic procedures, such a risk seems too high. The jury is still out.[20]

The management of acute penetrating eye injuries remains shrouded in debate, largely artificially for examination purposes. The conflict between the need to secure the airway, especially if the patient is not fasted and the case is urgent, and the need to prevent any loss of contents of the globe due to sudden rises in intraocular pressure is more rationally resolved with the recently released agents. One choice lies in using a potent opioid such as alfentanil or remifentanil immediately after administration of the induction agent to prevent rises in IOP and the use of rapacuronium[21] or rocuronium to facilitate endotracheal intubation*. Alternatively, suxamethonium can still be used, but with a priming dose of a non-depolarising muscle relaxant prior to induction.[22] In all cases full preoxygenation and cricoid pressure are mandatory.

The very unfit patient with severe respiratory failure has been thought of as too ill for a general anaesthetic. The ability to provide intravenous anaesthesia, profound but evanescent analgesia and minimal muscle relaxation whilst protecting their airway enables safe surgery to be performed. Recovery in the sitting position, with the improvement in oxygenation, further improves outcome. Oxygenation on the postoperative night is independent of whether a local or general anaesthetic is used.[23] Patients no longer need to be denied general anaesthesia.

Postoperative Care

The majority of ophthalmic procedures are performed on a day-care basis, and the return to a 'street-ready' condition is very important. The modern anaesthetic agents allow recovery within much the same time frame as a local anaesthetic technique. The time to take oral fluids is much shorter if the historical technique of spraying local anaesthetic onto the larynx and vocal cords is avoided. Once the patient can close their glottis, they can partake of clear fluids. Analgesia is rarely required, but treatment of nausea and vomiting may be necessary. This is most troublesome in strabismus surgery and will usually require a multi-modal range of therapy.

Summary

The provision of safe operating conditions and optimal care of the patient, whatever their age or state of health, can be achieved under general anaesthesia. The limitations of some centres where there are inadequate facilities for safe general anaesthesia or where investment in modern integrated anaesthetic machines and monitors is lacking prevent some patients from having optimal care.

General anaesthesia remains the primary option for many ophthalmic procedures and for many patients. The drive to provide many procedures under local anaesthesia, especially with the improved safety of modern techniques, is entirely appropriate but does not detract from the need to train anaesthetists skilled in the administration of general anaesthesia for ophthalmic surgery.

---

* Rapacurium has been withdrawn from use in the USA because of concerns with bronchospasm, but it remains available in the rest of the world at present.

References

1   Wolf G, Lynch S, Berlin I. Intraocular surgery with general anesthesia. *Arch Ophthalmol.* 1975; 93:323–326.

2   Campbell DN, Lim M, Muir MK, O'Sullivan G, Falcon M, Fison P, Woods R. A prospective randomised study of local versus general anaesthesia for cataract surgery. *Anaesthesia.* 1993; 48:422–428.

3   Edge R, Navon S. Scleral perforation during retrobulbar and peribulbar anesthesia: risk factors and outcome in 50,000 consecutive injections. *J Cataract Refract Surg.* 1999; 25:1237–1244.

4   Bullock JD, Warwar RE, Green WR. Ocular explosion during cataract surgery: a clinical, histopathological, experimental, and biophysical study. *Trans Am Ophthalmol Soc.* 1998; 96:243–276.

5   Norregaard JC, Bernth-Petersen P, Bellan L, Alonso J, Black C, Dunn E, Andersen TF, Espallargues M, Anderson G. Intraoperative clinical practice and risk of early complications after cataract extraction in the United States, Canada, Denmark, and Spain. *Ophthalmology.* 1999; 106:42–48.

6   Tarbet KJ, Custer PL. External dacryocystorhinostomy. Surgical success, patient satisfaction, and economic cost. *Ophthalmology.* 1995; 102:1065–1070.

7   Suttner S, Boldt J. Low-flow anaesthesia. Does it have potential pharmacoeconomic consequences? *Pharmacoeconomics.* 2000; 17:585–590.

8   Suttner SW, Schmidt CC, Boldt J, Huttner I, Kumle B, Piper SN. Low-flow desflurane and sevoflurane anesthesia minimally affect hepatic integrity and function in elderly patients. *Anesth Analg.* 2000; 91:206–212.

9   Stabernack CR, Brown R, Laster MJ, Dudziak R, Eger E. Absorbents differ enormously in their capacity to produce compound A and carbon monoxide. *Anesth Analg.* 2000; 90:1428–1435.

10 Bailey JM. Context-sensitive half-times and other decrement times of inhaled anesthetics. *Anesth Analg.* 1997; 85:681–686.

11 Baum J, Sievert B, Stanke HG, Brauer K, Sachs G. Nitrous oxide free low-flow anesthesia. *Anaesthesiol Reanim.* 2000; 25:60–67.

12 Sutcliffe NP, Hyde R, Martay K. Use of 'Diprifusor' in anaesthesia for ophthalmic surgery. *Anaesthesia.* 1998; 53 Suppl 1:49–52.

13 Sneyd JR, Carr A, Byrom WD, Bilski AJ. A meta-analysis of nausea and vomiting following maintenance of anaesthesia with propofol or inhalational agents. *Eur J Anaesthesiol.* 1998; 15:433–445.

14 De Mey JC, Debrock M, Rolly G. Evaluation of the onset and intubation conditions of rocuronium bromide. *Eur J Anaesthesiol Suppl.* 1994; 9:37–40.

15 Simpson KH, Smith RJ, Davies LF. Comparison of the effects of atropine and glycopyrrolate on cognitive function following general anaesthesia. *Br J Anaesth.* 1987; 59:966–969.

16 van den Berg AA, Lambourne A, Clyburn PA. The oculo-emetic reflex. A rationalisation of postophthalmic anaesthesia vomiting. *Anaesthesia.* 1989; 44(2):110–117.

17 Ali-Melkkila T, Kanto J, Katevuo R. Tropisetron and metoclopramide in the prevention of postoperative nausea and vomiting. A comparative, placebo controlled study in patients undergoing ophthalmic surgery. *Anaesthesia.* 1996; 51(3):232–235.

18 Ascaso FJ, Ayala I, Carbonell P, Castro FJ, Palomar A. Prophylactic intravenous ondansetron in patients undergoing cataract extraction under general anesthesia. *Ophthalmologica.* 1997; 211:292–295.

19 Myint Y, Singh AK, Peacock JE, Padfield A. Changes in intra-ocular pressure during general anaesthesia. A comparison of spontaneous breathing through a laryngeal mask

with positive pressure ventilation through a tracheal tube. *Anaesthesia.* 1995; 50:126–129.

20   Sidaras G, Hunter JM. Is it safe to artificially ventilate a paralysed patient through the laryngeal mask? The jury is still out. *Brit J Anaesth.* 2001; 86:749–753.

21   Blobner M, Mirakhur RK, Wierda JM, Wright PM, Olkkola KT, Debaene B, Penderville P, Engback J, Riethergen H. Rapacuronium 2.0 or 2.5 mg kg^{-1} for rapid-sequence induction: comparison with succinylcholine 1.0 mg kg^{-1}. *Br J Anaesth.* 2000; 85:724–731.

22   Wang ML, Seiff SR, Drasner K. A comparison of visual outcome in open-globe repair: succinylcholine with D-tubocurarine vs nondepolarizing agents. *Ophthalmic Surgery* 1992; 23:746–751.

23   McCarthy GJ, Mirakhur RK, Elliott P. Postoperative oxygenation in the elderly following general or local anaesthesia for ophthalmic surgery. *Anaesthesia.* 1992; 47:1090–1092.

12

Anaesthesia for Vitreoretinal Surgery

Dr Robert W. Johnson

Anatomy, Physiology and Pathology of Vitreous

The total ocular volume is approximately 6.5 ml of which vitreous forms 80%. It is in intimate contact with the retina, ciliary body and much of the posterior capsule of the lens. Vitreous is composed of collagen and hyaluronic acid and consists of long collagen fibres and a proteoglycan matrix that gives vitreous its viscous character. Hyaluronic acid has an enormous affinity for water and 99% of vitreous by weight is water. Vitreous may separate from the retina without damage to the retina or visual impairment other than perhaps the annoyance of floaters. However, it may separate with some tenacious strands remaining attached to the retina resulting in retinal tearing. Liquid vitreous may then flow behind components of the retina leading to separation of its layers and retinal detachment with serious visual impairment. Similarly, vitreal strands may cause traction on retinal blood vessels resulting in vitreous haemorrhage. Proliferative vitreoretinopathy is akin to scar tissue forming and spreading within the vitreous cortex. Concentrations of matrix and collagen combine with clotted blood plasma that has leaked from retinal vessels. Visual impairment is then from a combination of the opacity of the scar tissue membrane, buckling of the retina and, sometimes, retinal detachment.

Scope of Surgery

Surgery for pathology involving the retina may require an approach from outside the globe applying instruments such as a cryoprobe or explants (bands or plombs), or from inside the globe through the vitreous cavity of the eye, or both. Such surgery may be undertaken for trauma involving a foreign body lodged in the vitreous, for consequences of systemic disease such as diabetes or Marfan's syndrome, for retinal detachment or for correction of complications of cataract surgery where part or all of the lens has become displaced posteriorly into the vitreous. Surgical relocation of areas of retina in macular degeneration is now undertaken. Vitrectomy may also form part of the management of tumours within the eye or infection. These patients frequently have very severe visual impairment prior to surgery and small improvements may make a vast difference to quality of life, as restoration of vision adequate to permit independent navigation is enormously worthwhile.

Retinal Detachment Surgery without Vitrectomy

The aim of surgery for retinal detachment is to re-attach the retina to the choroid by a combination of actions. During this procedure there is tissue dissection on the exterior of the globe to permit either a foam or silicone plomb/sponge or encircling band to be applied over the detachment site to indent or buckle the sclera towards the detached retina. The precise means by which buckling achieves its results is multifactorial and a clear description is provided by Charles and Small.[1] The cryoprobe is applied to encourage an inflammatory response, 'welding' the retinal layers to the buckled wall of the globe. In addition, subretinal fluid may be aspirated with a fine needle from the external surface and/or a gas bubble may be injected. There is significant manipulation of the globe and tissue dissection, resulting in considerable painful stimulus both intraoperatively and postoperatively.

When a detachment is incomplete, so called 'macula on', some surgeons will wish to carry out surgery as an emergency, although most cases can be delayed to permit proper preparation for safe anaesthesia. Because of the significant painful stimulus, such surgery is often undertaken with general anaesthesia (GA). Good quality local anaesthesia (LA) is satisfactory but intraoperative sub-Tenon's augmentation of the block is often necessary in prolonged cases. Postoperative pain may be significant. A study at the Wills Eye Hospital in Philadelphia, USA, reported that retrobulbar irrigation with 0.75% bupivacaine at the end of surgery reduces the requirement for parenteral analgesia postoperatively.[2]

Vitrectomy

The vitrector consists of an intraocular hollow probe incorporating a tiny cutting instrument at the tip that can operate at various frequencies to fragment by snipping small pieces of the viscous vitreous, which are then aspirated via the lumen of the tube. Light can be applied to the operative area via a fine fibre-optic probe. Sharp dissecting instruments, such as scissors and picks, may also be introduced through small puncture holes through the sclera at the pars plana. Some instruments contain an integral fibre-optic light source. As vitreous is removed, a similar volume of balanced salt solution (BSS) enters the eye to replace it. Electrocautery and laser coagulation may also be applied from within the vitreous cavity. Tissues are sometimes delineated by vital staining with indocyanine green.

In some situations, an inert, low-solubility gas, such as sulphur hexafluoride (SF_6) or C_3F_8, frequently diluted with air, is injected into the cavity previously occupied by vitreous to cause a tamponade of the retina onto the choroid. (The implications of the presence of intravitreal gas are discussed below.) Alternatively, silicone oil may be left in the vitreous cavity for removal at a later date. Heavy fluid may be injected to facilitate removal of some foreign bodies by flotation or to provide tamponade during surgery without the need to place the patient in an inconvenient posture.

Spectrum of Patients

Patients of all ages may require vitreoretinal (VR) surgery but the majority are adults. A strong association of retinal pathology with diabetes dictates that the anaesthetist must contend with the many systemic complications of that disease and the drugs used in its management. As these patients may exhibit multiple systemic illnesses, anaesthetic considerations must take into account both surgical and disease-related issues.

Special Surgical Requirements

Retinal surgery varies in duration and it is not always clear at the start of a case how long it may take. An anaesthetic technique that permits flexibility is wise. The degree of surgical stimulus also varies significantly — that produced by the intraocular component of vitrectomy is mild with the exception of laser application, whilst external work, especially application of the cryoprobe, leads to significant stimulation. The short more painful episodes may take place towards the end of surgery and it is most unwise to allow the depth of anaesthesia or analgesic component to wear thin until surgery is completed. Finally, the surgical episode frequently finishes with examination of the contralateral eye and may involve application of the cryoprobe to it.

VR surgery frequently takes place in a darkened room, and the anaesthetist's vision may be further impaired at times by the required wearing of filter spectacles or goggles to protect against laser exposure to the eye. Availability of a torch/flashlight to allow record keeping, monitoring and personal safety becomes important.

Intraocular Pressure (IOP)

IOP control is important and is under the control of the anaesthetist at the start and finish of surgery. During the bulk of the operation, the surgeon and his vitrectomy equipment will override our normal considerations. However, it is sensible to maintain normal homeostasis throughout the operation as choroidal blood flow responds to changes in blood pressure and carbon dioxide tension. IOP will also change with increases or decreases in the volume of an injected gas bubble that may result from the use of nitrous oxide (N_2O).

An important difference between vitrectomy and other ocular surgery is the requirement in some cases for injection of a gas mixture that will remain in the posterior chamber for several days. The problems related to the presence of a gas within a cavity, the lining of which is perfused by blood, are not unique to eye surgery and are well known in the cases of gas within other perfused cavities such as the pleura, the middle ear, or the gut. The choice of gas between SF_6, C_3F_8 and C_4F_8, and its percentage mixture in air, will depend on how long the surgeon wishes it to remain before absorption. The anaesthetic significance lies in the low solubility and diffusion characteristics of these gases and the dynamic relationship with nitrous oxide. Sulphur hexafluoride, and C_3F_8 and C_4F_8 are very insoluble in water and SF_6 has an Ostwald solubility coefficient of 0.004 (1.16) compared with oxygen 0.022 (2.2), nitrogen 0.014 (2.01) and nitrous oxide 0.468 (2.6) — diffusion coefficients appear in brackets after solubility coefficients. When injected into the vitreous cavity the more soluble nitrous oxide from the blood and tissues will diffuse into the bubble much more rapidly than the SF_6 can diffuse out. There will be an increase in the volume of the bubble and a secondary increase in pressure on surrounding structures. Discontinuing nitrous oxide administration reverses this process reducing the volume of the bubble. Air alone produces a bubble that is absorbed within a few hours because of the ready absorption of nitrogen and oxygen into the surrounding tissues and circulation.

Increases in volume/pressure may jeopardise circulation to the retina, whilst decreases will negate the intended tamponade effect. Stinson and Donlon produced a mathematical model to predict the time course and extent of the volume/pressure effects of nitrous oxide on the injected bubble.[3] They calculated that intravitreal injection of SF_6/air mixture in the presence of inhalational administration of 70% nitrous oxide would produce a significant expansion of the bubble within 60 minutes. The less soluble the injected gas mixture the greater the expansion. Depending on the compliance of the eye, pressure would increase as a result. Animal work suggests rises in IOP of 15 to 20 mm Hg are possible — the consequent reduction of the perfusion of the retina could be critical. The alveolar concentration of nitrous oxide decreases by 90% within 10 minutes of its withdrawal from the inspired gas mixture (assuming adequate fresh gas flow) and bubble volume regains the injected figure within about 20 minutes. The expansion in the presence of 70% N_2O may be up to 300% of its original value.

Nitrous oxide may be totally avoided or alternatively may be withdrawn at least 15 minutes before the gas is injected. Volatile anaesthetic agents in oxygen alone or in an oxygen/air mixture exert little effect on the intravitreal bubble. Air/oxygen mixtures are preferable to 100% oxygen as a ventilatory gas because of the possible adverse effects of pure oxygen on retinal circulation and of the increased risk of postoperative atelectasis. Because the surgeon cannot always decide if intravitreal injection will be necessary before the start of surgery, adaptation of technique may become necessary. The bubble may remain as an entity for 10 days, so further anaesthesia within this time should avoid the use of N_2O.

Choice of Anaesthetic Technique

Traditionally in the UK vitreoretinal surgery has been undertaken with GA largely because of the longer duration of surgery. Certainly comfort of the patient as a whole may be more problematic than comfort of the eye. In the USA LA is more common and there is a marked trend in the same direction in the UK. With experience on the part of the theatre team and a confident and calm ambience, the procedure performed under LA can be a positive experience for the patient, avoiding many of the less desirable facets of GA. Local anaesthesia is especially advantageous when very early posturing following gas bubble injection is required as in the case of retinal reloca- tion surgery for macular degeneration. In the absence of relative contraindications to general anaesthesia, the choice of anaesthetic technique should be tailored to the preferences of the patient, the surgeon and the anaesthetist.

Patient assessment should be identical for local or general anaesthesia.[4] Preoperative fasting is recommended for all patients undergoing elective retinal sur- gery because of the unpredictable duration of the procedure, irrespective of the anaesthetic technique.

General Anaesthesia

Control of the airway and intraocular pressure are cornerstones of anaesthesia for VR surgery. Airway protection by an endotracheal tube or a laryngeal mask airway (LMA) is the subject of current debate, and either choice may be appropriate. A com- plete discussion may be found in Chapter 11. The author prefers to use a LMA only if there are no contraindications, maintaining a very low threshold for the use of an endotracheal tube.

A satisfactory GA technique must provide autonomic stability, maintain choroidal blood flow and IOP and ensure a rapid and complete recovery. Immobility of the patient during surgery is of paramount importance. The condition of the patient, the skills of the anaesthetist and the expected duration of surgery dictate the choice of anaesthetic agents, both for induction and maintenance.

Combination Techniques

A reduction in requirement for perioperative systemic analgesia, postoperative pain relief and reduction of PONV[5] all make perioperative LA block advantageous.

The author prefers to perform a nasal canthal (medial compartment) peribulbar (extraconal) block because of the enhanced anaesthesia that it offers for adnexal structures. In an eye of unknown dimensions this is probably the safest pathway to the extraconal space. Others favour the sub-Tenon's route of administration. For pro- longed surgery, a supplement given by the surgeon by the sub-Tenon's route towards the end of the operation prolongs the effect.

The author prefers to insert the block after induction and safe control of the air- way, but others feel this is better performed prior to induction of anaesthesia.

Oculocardiac Reflex (OCR)

The extent to which the globe is manipulated during VR surgery varies, but is great- est during indirect ophthalmoscopy and application of explants for scleral buckling.

The stretching of the extraocular muscles may precipitate this reflex as described in Chapter 3. Orbital blocks usually, but not always, attenuate the reflex. Prophylactic anticholinergic drugs are also variably effective unless used in large doses that may produce unwanted cardiac effects.

There is no alternative to vigilant observation with remedial treatment when indicated. Firstly, the surgeon is enthusiastically invited to discontinue the provocative action, and, second, an anticholinergic drug is given intravenously. Asystole can occur.

Temperature Regulation and IV Fluids

The duration of the procedure, ambient temperature and humidity of the operating area, age of the patient and bodily build will determine the extent of heat loss during surgery. Temperature monitoring is highly recommended, and active warming may be necessary during the procedure.

Fluid deficits are negligible and solely related to insensible losses and fasting. High volume fluid therapy should be avoided to prevent bladder distension or precipitating congestive cardiac failure in compromised patients.

Local Anaesthesia

Retrobulbar (intraconal), peribulbar (extraconal) and sub-Tenon's techniques have all been used with success: the choice should depend on the ability of the technique to satisfy the required conditions for VR surgery with a high degree of safety as well as the experience of the anaesthetist.

It is reasonable to request that biometry be undertaken in these cases to offer guidance to the anaesthetist regarding axial length. In the absence of biometry knowing the patient's spectacle prescription is helpful because highly myopic patients tend to have very long eyes. In the absence of reliable information, it is necessary to assume a long eye and tailor the block accordingly.

Prolonged surgery places a number of demands on the patient and anaesthetist. Apart from comfort of the eye and good surgical conditions, it is necessary to keep the rest of the patient's body comfortable. This requires careful positioning on the operating table or reclining chair, padding of bony areas and a pillow placed under the knees to relieve strain on knees, hips and spine. One should be able to control temperature, and a forced warm air device is one way to achieve this. In our institution the patient is allowed a 'wriggle break' every 30 minutes or so. The surgeon removes his instruments from the eye and raises the microscope slightly following which the patient is invited to move their limbs and back to restore comfort. This procedure should be rehearsed with the patient before the start of surgery. Music should be inoffensive to the patient and operating room team!

Knight et al.[6] reported an observational audit of 178 patients, which showed that most of the discomfort during surgery was from the operating table, and that most of their patients would choose a LA for further surgery.

Whilst many anaesthetists prefer a sub-Tenon's block,[7–9] the author prefers to perform a peribulbar (extraconal) block*. For prolonged surgery, the surgeon may easily reinforce the block with additional local anaesthetic introduced into the sub-Tenon's space.

Sedation may be desirable for some patients but should always leave the patient awake and able to communicate. The author rarely exceeds 1 mg of midazolam in 0.5 mg increments and 20 mg propofol in 5 mg increments. Others favour the use of small boluses of narcotic such as alfentanil. This can be useful in the patient with a cough. If coughing arises during surgery for the first time, the presence of congestive cardiac failure should be considered.

Postoperative Care

Postoperative Nausea and Vomiting (PONV)

Postoperative nausea and vomiting, immediate and delayed, are notorious accompaniments of VR surgery. It is very unpleasant for patients and may even prejudice the outcome of surgery, for example by delaying important posturing following intravitreal gas injection. Van den Berg[10] reported results of a study of 607 patients including children and adults. Early and delayed PONV were identified, the former occurring within minutes of the completion of surgery. Early PONV was noted in 10% of patients after squint surgery, 2.7% after orbital surgery and 1.8% after ocular operations other than squint correction. Delayed PONV incidences were 57% after squint operations, 23% for orbital surgery and 18% in ocular non-squint patients.[10] An oculo-emetic reflex is suggested which may be initiated by manipulation of and trauma to the globe. The precise nervous pathway is uncertain (see Chapter 3).

A history of PONV is always of concern because it may suggest resistance to preventive measures, may increase patient apprehension, and may foreshadow the possibility of further problems.

The literature provides contradictory advice on management and anaesthetists tend to learn by experience subtle techniques that significantly reduce the problem.

---

* The author uses 25 mm 25 or 27 G needles and warmed 0.75% bupivacaine or L-bupivacaine with hyalase 10 IU per ml. A pre-injection of approximately 1ml of 0.2% warmed lidocaine in Balanced Salt Solution (BSS) as advised by Hustead renders the technique virtually painless. For prolonged surgery with extraocular components, I use three insertion points. The first two are as for cataract surgery, inferotemporal (at the lateral point of the inferior rim of the orbit) and medial compartment from the blind pit where the caruncle meets the medial canthus, and superotemporal insertion. This latter point is chosen because of the greater safety of this route to the mid-orbit compared with the obsolete and inappropriate superonasal insertion that inevitably brings the needle into close contact with vulnerable muscle and blood vessels. The third insertion point is used because of the experience of many VR anaesthetists that optimal anaesthesia in the upper quadrants often fails without it. With good anatomical knowledge and experience this is not a difficult or hazardous addition to the routine extraconal block. The superotemporal insertion is through skin not conjunctiva. The brain is separated from the needle by bone that can easily be pierced by a needle. The total volume of injectate is adjusted to take account of the patient's orbit, size and frailty.

The author's favoured technique involves the intravenous use of the 5-HT$_3$ inhibitors, (ondanstron 4 mg or granisetron 1 mg), and dexamethasone 4 to 6 mg intraoperatively with provision of analgesia by LA block performed either before the start or towards the end of surgery, or both if surgery is prolonged. This combination is best administered towards the end of the operation. The place of acupuncture is uncertain.

Patient Positioning

The purpose of creating a gas bubble is to tamponade the retinal break and to provide a surface tension barrier to the passage of fluid into the subretinal space. To optimise the position of the bubble over the intended site, the patient will need to adopt prescribed postures for a significant proportion of the time for several days. The posture should be adopted as soon as possible after surgery and this favours the use of LA techniques, because postoperative nausea and vomiting and/or delayed recovery will hinder this important aspect of treatment.

Postoperative Analgesia

In the absence of persistent local anaesthesia postoperative pain can be significant and difficult to manage. Long-acting local anaesthetics given perioperatively can be of great benefit. In the hospitalised patient, continuous local anaesthetic techniques have been described.[11,12] NSAIDS are also of benefit in the absence of contraindications. Opiates, including long-acting oral preparations, will sometimes be required, particularly following buckling procedures. Additional antiemetics may be required when these are used.

Postoperative Advice

When intravitreal gas has been injected, patients should be warned about the effects of further anaesthesia over the next few weeks with respect to nitrous oxide and the effects of changed atmospheric pressure during aircraft flights. Most commercial aircraft are pressurised to 3000 m and this will cause the gas bubble to expand to about double its intended volume with a proportional increase in IOP, which may lead to retinal ischaemia or even globe rupture.

References

1   Charles S, Small KM. Pathogenesis and repair of retinal detachment. In: Easty DL, Sparrow JM, editors. *Oxford Textbook of Ophthalmology*, Vol 2. Oxford Medical Publications, Oxford, 1999. pp 1261–1272.
2   Duker JA, Nielsen J, Vander JF, Rosenstein RB, Benson WE. Retrobulbar bupivacaine irrigation for postoperative pain after sclera buckling surgery: a prospective study. *Ophthalmology.* 1991; 98:514.
3   Stinson TW, Donlon JV. Interaction of intraocular air and sulphur hexafluoride with nitrous oxide: a computer simulation. *Anesthesiology.* 1982; 56:385–388.
4   Report of the Joint Working Party on Anaesthesia in Ophthalmic Surgery: Royal College of Anaesthetists and College of Ophthalmologists, London, March 1993.

5   Gottfreothdottir MS, Gislason I, Stefansson E, Sigurjonsdottir S, Nielsen CN. Effects of retrobulbar bupivacaine on post-operative pain and nausea in retinal detachment surgery. *Acta Ophthalmol.* 1993; 71:544–547.

6   Knight HML, Newsom RB, Canning CR, Luff AJ, Wainwright AC. BOAS Annual Scientific Meeting, Bristol, England, June 2000. Abstract 12.

7   Mein CE, Woodcock MG. Local anesthesia for vitreoretinal surgery. *Retina.* 1990; 10:47–49.

8   Kwok AK, Van Newkirk MR, Lam DS, Fan DS. Sub-Tenon's anesthesia in vitreoretinal surgery: a needleless technique. *Retina.* 1999; 19:291–296.

9   Stevens JD, Franks WA, Orr G, Leaver PK, Cooling RJ. Four-quadrant local anaesthesia technique for vitreoretinal surgery. *Eye.* 1992; 6:583–586.

10 Van den Berg AA, Lambourne A, Clayburn PA. The oculo-emetic reflex, a rationalization of post ophthalmic anaesthesia vomiting. *Anaesthesia.* 1989; 44:110–117.

11 Bernard JM, Hommeril JL. Prolonged peribulbar anaesthesia with indwelling catheter: a preliminary report of 217 cases. *Br J Anaesth.* 1997; 78:81–82.

12 Jonas JB, Hemmerling TM, Budde WM, Dinkel M. Postoperative analgesia by re-injections of local anesthetic through an indwelling retrobulbar catheter. *Am J Ophthalmol.* 2000; 129:54–58.

13

Anaesthesia Management of Patients with Uveal Tract Melanoma

Dr Steven Gayer

Introduction

Ocular Tumours

Melanoma is a potentially lethal disease that has many forms and presentations. Primary ocular melanoma is particularly insidious. It is frequently painless and otherwise asymptomatic in its early stages. It is often first suspected upon routine ophthalmologic examination. Left untreated or undiagnosed, it can metastasise and be fatal. Whilst there are a variety of orbital and ocular tumours that can arise in the population, melanoma of the uveal tract is the most common primary eye cancer encountered in adults in the United States. Ophthalmologists employ a number of diagnostic methods and clinical interventions in the treatment of ocular melanoma. The traditional means of therapy, ocular enucleation, is being supplemented to some extent by new therapies such as surgical implantation of radioactive materials. The perioperative concerns, anaesthetic implications, and management of patients with primary uveal tract melanoma differ markedly for patients undergoing enucleation versus surgical radiation therapy. Orbital tumours may be primary or secondary, benign or malignant, intraocular or extraocular, and so forth. Secondary tumours may result from metastatic spread from distant locations or via direct extension of an extraocular tumour into the eye. The latter is quite rare.

Ocular cancer is classified by histology and anatomic location. Abnormal growth in the anterior chamber and trabecular meshwork is most commonly the result of melanoma invading from the uveal tract. Rarely, lymphoma occurs in the vitreous. The sclera is infrequently the target of primary neoplastic involvement, whilst the retina is the site of the most common paediatric primary eye neoplasm, retinoblastoma.[1]

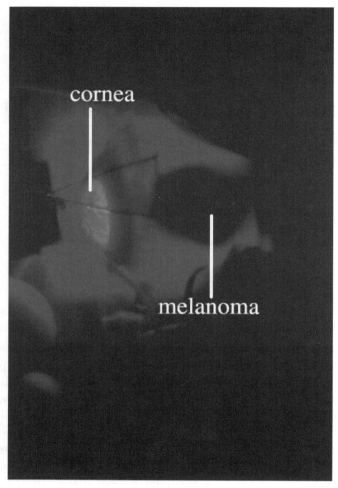

Fig. 1.   Transillumination of an in-situ choroidal melanoma. Antonio Cubillas, Bascom Palmer Eye
          Institute, Department of Photography.

Retinoblastoma is responsible for almost 1% of all paediatric cancer deaths and
accounts for nearly 3% of all childhood cancers. Approximately 40% of children
have bilateral tumours. The presenting symptoms usually include leukocoria and strabismus. The genetic basis for retinoblastoma has been identified as a lack or malfunction of a gene on the long arm of chromosome thirteen, whose usual function is
to prevent formation of neoplasias in healthy individuals. This gene was the first
allelomorph with tumour-suppressing function to be differentiated.[2,3] In adults, the
most frequently encountered orbital tumours are metastatic lesions to the eye and the
surrounding orbit. The most common primary eye cancer is melanoma of the uveal
tract, particularly the choroid and ciliary body. In the USA, the incidence of uveal
melanoma is six to eight cases per million people per year. The tumour is rarely

detected in the paediatric population. Uveal tract melanoma primarily affects adults sixty to seventy years of age; however, there is also an enhanced incidence in the third decade of life.[4]

Uveal Tract Melanoma

The globe itself is comprised of three distinct layers, the sclera, the uveal tract, and the retina. The sclera consists of tough, fibrous materials that serve to provide intrinsic structural support and rigidity for the globe. Anteriorly, the sclera becomes the clear cornea, which allows light to penetrate into the eye to ultimately reach the innermost layer, the retina. Posteriorly, the sclera is continuous with the dural sheath surrounding the optic nerve.[5,6]

The uveal tract comprises the middle layer of the eye. It consists of three sections: the choroid, the ciliary body, and the iris (Figure 2). In marked contrast to the rather avascular scleral layer, the uveal tract contains a plethora of vessels. In the posterior portion of the globe, the choroid lies between the sclera and the retina. At the optic nerve, it is continuous with the pia and arachnoid layers. There is a potential space between the sclera and choroid, called the suprachoroidal space. The choroid itself consists of three distinct layers, one of which, the choriocapillaris, provides a conduit for transport of nutrients to the outer part of the retina via a plexus of arterioles and capillaries.

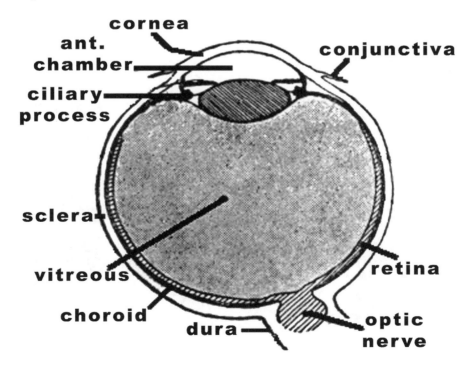

Fig. 2. Diagram of ocular anatomy.

The ciliary body is a direct anterior extension of the choroid. It is divided into two parts: the anterior pars plicata and the posterior pars plana. The pars plicata contains the ciliary processes. The ciliary body has dual function. It produces aqueous humour and makes accommodation possible by using its internal musculature to alter the shape of the lens. The third portion of the uveal tract is the iris, which is continuous with the ciliary body. It consists of a ring of pigmented tissue surrounding the pupil and serves to regulate the degree of light allowed into the eye.[5,6]

Due to its highly vascular nature, the choroid is a frequent site for metastasis of extraocular tumours. Metastatic spread to the choroid is the most commonly encountered intraocular tumour in adults. There are approximately two thousand new cases diagnosed per year in the USA. Primary tumours arise most often from breast, lung, or prostate cancer. Metastatic lesions may be multiple and occur simultaneously in both eyes.[1]

In contrast to metastatic spread of cancer to the uveal tract, primary melanoma usually affects just one eye and is singular in nature (Figure 3). The disease affects both genders equally, with greater incidence in individuals of fair complexion. Caucasians have up to a tenfold greater risk than African-Americans. There may be a genetic predisposition to ocular melanoma and some clinicians postulate that cigarette smoking is also a risk factor.[1,4,7]

Presenting symptoms depend on the location and size of the tumour. Large lesions near the macula may produce visual changes early in the progress of the disease whilst

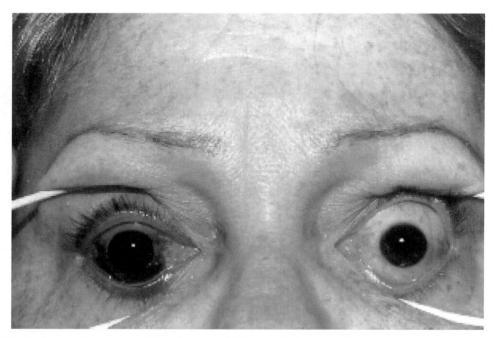

Fig. 3.   Large primary choroidal melanoma of right eye. Left eye unaffected. Antonio Cubillas, Bascom Palmer Eye Institute, Department of Photography.

ciliary body melanomas can expand behind the iris and may fail to be discovered until very late. Uveal tract melanomas usually do not produce early symptoms.[4,7]

Prognosis is dependent upon histopathology and size. Spindle-shaped melanoma cells have a better prognosis than epithelioid-shaped cells (Figures 4 and 5). Most uveal tract melanomas have a mixture of both cell types and thus an intermediate prognosis. Smaller masses are less likely than larger tumours to have metastasised and thus imply a more favourable prognosis.[1,4,7,8]

The Armed Forces Institute of Pathology examined melanoma-affected eyes after enucleation and reported a distribution of approximately 30% small tumours, 40% medium sized tumours, and 30% large sized primary uveal tract melanomas. The Collaborative Ocular Melanoma Study has found a similar distribution in in-situ eyes. Figure 1 above depicts an eye with a large choroidal melanoma.[7,8]

The five-year mortality of treated uveal tract melanoma is 50% for large melanomas, 30% for medium sized tumours, and up to 12% in small choroidal melanomas. More recently, a 6% five-year mortality from small choroidal melanomas has been reported.[9] Ocular melanomas tend to metastasise preferentially to liver, lung, and bone. In those individuals who have a metastatic spread of uveal tract melanoma, evidence of malignancy is often diagnosed within 2 to 4 years after definitive treatment. The median survival rate once metastatic disease is found is 6 to 9 months.[1,4,7,9]

Initial diagnosis depends upon a careful history and indirect ophthalmoscopy. Once suspected, other investigations may include slit-lamp examination, fluorescein angiography, direct fundus photography, ultrasound, CT scan and magnetic reso-

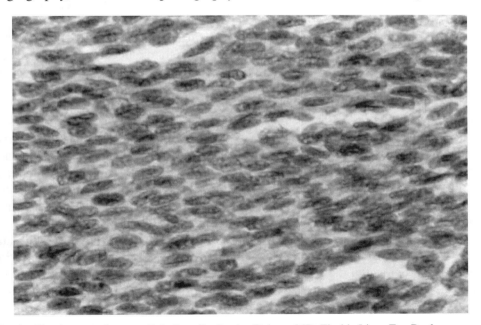

Fig. 4. Uveal tract melanoma: Spindle cells. Sandor Dubovy MD, Florida Lions Eye Bank.

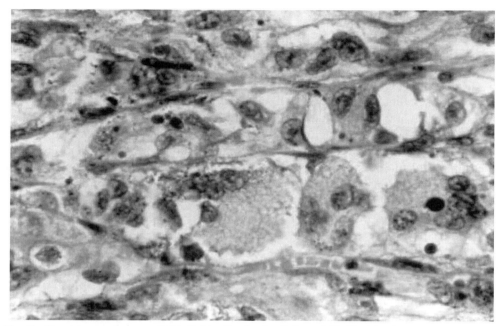

Fig. 5.   Uveal tract melanoma: Epithelioid cells. Sandor Dubovy MD, Florida Lions Eye Bank.

nance imaging (MRI). It is important to note that the diagnosis is based upon these indirect tests and not by direct biopsy of suspected lesions. Surgical biopsy of an ocular mass may result in compromise of vision and metastasis of tumour.[1,7]

Once a diagnosis of choroidal or ciliary body melanoma is made, a search for any metastatic tumour is important, because patients with evidence of metastasis have such a poor prognosis. This information will determine the choice of treatment for the patient.

Treatment

Enucleation remains the traditional method of treatment for primary uveal tract melanoma; however, alternative methods of treatment are being used before such destructive surgery. Radiotherapy, either by external beam radiation or episcleral application of radioactive plaque, may be utilized as alternative therapy to enucleation. Other alternative therapies include proton beam irradiation, cryotherapy, photocoagulation, chemotherapy, and immunotherapy.[1,10,11]

The appropriate therapy for primary choroidal and ciliary body tumours is the subject of an ongoing debate amongst ophthalmologists. Proponents of enucleation believe that removal of the globe is the only definitive and curative treatment for this disease. They argue that alternative therapies unnecessarily risk patients' lives in order to preserve vision. Advocates of alternative therapies such as episcleral radioactive plaque application point out that such treatment may preserve both the globe and

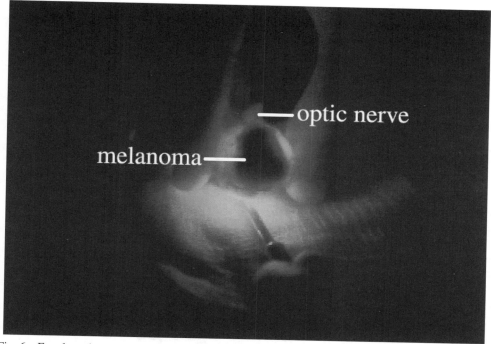

Fig. 6. Enucleated eye with large choroidal melanoma. Note the thick, stout optic nerve. Antonio Cubillas, Bascom Palmer Eye Institute, Department of Photography.

vision, and result in enhanced quality of life without increased morbidity. A few ophthalmologists are even of the opinion that surgical manipulation of the globe during enucleation may result in metastases and increased morbidity. The majority of large and medium-sized uveal tract primary melanomas are treated by enucleation (see Figure 6). However, most ophthalmologists do not actively treat small choroidal tumours until there is evidence of change in the nature of the mass. Some, however, believe that initiation of therapy early on may ultimately result in overall improved survival.[7–13] Whichever treatment modality is ultimately proven more beneficial, the anaesthetist must be prepared to encounter patients in the operating room with the same disease undergoing vastly different surgical procedures.[4,14]

Episcleral radioactive plaque application consists of placing a plaque embedded with radioactive seeds in proximity to the melanoma. The plaque is shielded with gold on one side, so that the radiation is directed at the lesion, with minimal radioactive exposure to surrounding unaffected tissue (Figures 7 and 8).

Perioperative Anaesthesia Management of Patients with Uveal Tract Melanoma

Enucleation

Patients with primary intraocular melanoma who elect to have enucleation come to the operating room anticipating a single, definitive operation. In some countries, the

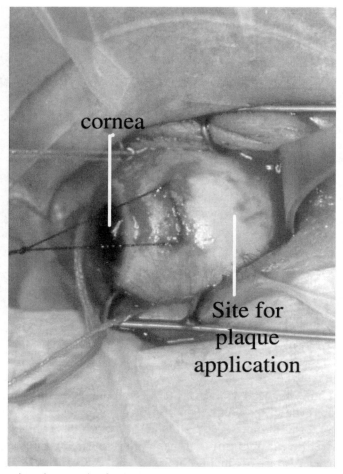

Fig. 7. Intraoperative photograph of sclera prepared for radioactive plaque implantation. Antonio
Cubillas, Bascom Palmer Eye Institute, Department of Photography.

majority of these cases are scheduled as ambulatory procedures with the patient discharged from the facility within a few hours following surgery, whilst in others
overnight stay is advocated. Patients are frequently anxious preoperatively since the
eye to be removed often retains visual function, the diagnosis of cancer has been
established by indirect means, and there is the ultimate potential of life-threatening
secondary spread of the tumour. Anxiolytic medication prior to surgery may be warranted. Benzodiazepines are the agents of choice and may be administered orally or
intravenously.

    Ocular enucleation can be accomplished using either general or regional anaes-
thesia, although there are issues involved in the selection of the appropriate type of
anaesthesia. The majority of patients with primary uveal tract melanoma are between
60 and 70 years of age, and the anaesthetic considerations for elderly patients are
numerous. They include age-related changes in cardiopulmonary, renal, hepatic, and

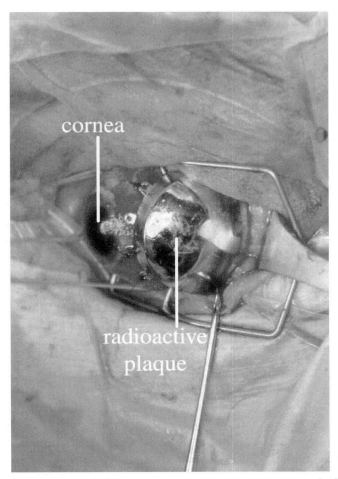

Fig. 8. Intraoperative photograph depicting implanted radioactive plaque. Antonio Cubillas, Bascom Palmer Eye Institute, Department of Photography.

central nervous system functions. Concomitant disease such as osteo-arthritis, diabetes, hypertension, and coronary artery disease may affect the selection of anaesthesia technique and/or medications.[15,16] The minimum alveolar concentration of anaesthetic agents declines with increasing age such that there are diminished dose requirements of anaesthetic needed to induce and maintain general anaesthesia in the elderly.[17,18] The airway can be secured during general anaesthesia either by using a laryngeal mask airway or an endotracheal tube. Inhalational or total intravenous techniques are appropriate for this procedure.

The oculocardiac reflex (see Chapter 3) is commonly encountered during enucleation under general anaesthesia. It manifests as a sudden bradycardia or even an asystolic cardiac arrest. Hypoxemia, hypercarbia, or light levels of general anaesthesia may exacerbate the bradycardic response.[19] The management of this reflex relies on stopping the precipitating stimulus — surgery and traction — and the administration of an anticholinergic agent. Atropine should be avoided in the elderly because of its adverse effects on the central nervous system. Local anaesthetic instilled by the surgeon after induction of general anaesthesia may inhibit the afferent portion of the oculocardiac reflex and prevent or attenuate any abrupt bradycardia due to ocular manipulation. Paradoxically, a block may precipitate an oculocardiac reflex response. Intraoperative local anaesthetic may also reduce postoperative discomfort.[20,21] The oculocardiac reflex may display tachyphylaxis, the bradycardic response fatiguing with repeated stimuli.[22]

Postoperative nausea and vomiting after general anaesthesia for enucleation of a cancerous eye may occur, perhaps as the result of the oculo-emetic reflex.[23]

Regional anaesthesia (with sedation) remains an alternative to general anaesthesia for patients undergoing ocular enucleation. Regional anaesthesia has to provide a dense motor and sensory block of suitable duration. The density of a regional anaesthetic block may be affected by the concentration and volume of local anaesthetic administered as well as by the additives employed. The addition of epinephrine will prolong and intensify analgesia and produces vasoconstriction that may diminish intraoperative bleeding.

The technique for the regional anaesthesia depends on using a high volume of concentrated local anaesthetic, usually as a peribulbar injection. Supplemental injections may be required.

One of the principal benefits of general anaesthesia is amnesia. Intraoperative awareness and recall are not important issues for patients undergoing cataract extraction and lens implantation; however, they are key factors in enucleation surgery under regional anaesthesia. One seeks to prevent any intraoperative recall or pain, particularly when the thick, stout optic nerve is transected as the last step prior to removing the globe from the orbit (see Chapters 8 and 14). Deep sedation is contraindicated for most ophthalmologic operations since potential abrupt head movements associated with changing levels of anaesthetic depth or responses by the anaesthetist or patient to airway obstruction may jeopardize the eye. The need for amnesia and ablation of awareness outweighs these factors for patients undergoing ocular enucleation, since jeopardising the eye is not an issue.

The Collaborative Ocular Melanoma Study[12] reported postoperative complications of large choroidal melanoma enucleation surgery without distinction as to type of anaesthesia. The most frequent postoperative problems were pain, nausea/vomiting, and haemorrhage. Cardiovascular and pulmonary complications, urinary retention, and fever may also occur. The reported incidences of pain (2%) and nausea/vomiting (<1%) are low and may be due to the fact that all reporting of data was done by the operating surgeons, without consulting anaesthesia or nursing personnel.[24]

Episcleral Plaque Radiotherapy

There are a number of distinctions between ocular enucleation and the surgical placement of a radioactive plaque for treatment of intraocular uveal tract melanoma. The former is usually accomplished as a single procedure, whilst the latter requires two operations. The duration of surgery for both the application of the radioactive plaque and its later removal is brief. As the pathology is intraocular, not intraorbital, there is no disease-related contraindication to regional anaesthesia. In contrast to ocular enucleation, the great majority of patients undergoing episcleral plaque radiotherapy receive conduction anaesthesia. In our experience, severe claustrophobia is the most commonly encountered indication for general anaesthesia. If the procedure is accomplished using general anaesthesia, it is necessary to avoid hypoventilation, since hypercarbia will induce increased blood flow to the vessel-rich choroid and make surgery more formidable.[5]

Due to extensive surgical manipulation of the globe in the course of implantation of the episcleral plaque, topical anaesthesia is not a feasible option. Peribulbar or sub-Tenon's injection of local anaesthetics is appropriate. Postoperatively, there may be an increased incidence of nausea/vomiting secondary to external pressure on the globe by the protective lead-lined shield placed at the conclusion of surgery. Administration of antiemetic preoperatively as well as postoperatively is helpful.

Anaesthesia for the second surgical procedure, removal of the radioactive episcleral plaque, begins with the preoperative interview. Whilst in the hospital, patients are restricted to a private room, their used linens remain with them, and their trash is not removed. This policy is adhered to in order to minimize other people's radiation exposure and to assure that no radioactive materials are lost, since there is the theoretical possibility that a radioactive iodine seed may become dislodged from the plaque and be displaced outside the eye. Patients frequently express frustration from the restriction of free movement during the three days of inpatient status. Anaesthesia and other personnel must express appropriate empathy.

Patients undergoing surgical removal of a plaque have the equivalent of a space-occupying intraorbital mass consisting of the radioactive plaque itself, surgical materials, and local tissue engorgement. Tissue engorgement is a response to the recent surgical manipulation, foreign body implantation, and radiation. This expansion of intraorbital mass markedly reduces the free volume within the orbit, thus diminishing the potential space for local anaesthetics. Sub-Tenon's blocks are less effective since it is difficult to thread the blunt cannula posteriorly, and local anaesthetics tend to reflux forward. Peribulbar block requires higher volumes of local anaesthetic agent, but even minimal volume may be very difficult to inject.

The author performs a low-volume retrobulbar block in those patients returning to the surgical suite for removal of a radioactive plaque. The incidence of bradycardia due to the oculocardiac reflex is high. The quality of analgesia may be poor and often needs to be supplemented with intravenous and intraorbital medications. In addition to sedatives and/or opioids, intravenous propofol is a useful adjunct due to its short duration of action and antiemetic properties. Its propensity for inducing apnoea and bradycardia must be noted. The removal of the plaque usually takes less than twenty minutes.

Occasionally, local blocks may fail with inadequate analgesia and general anaesthesia is then necessary. Appropriate fasting should have been observed to allow such a change of plan.

Another method to accomplish and maintain regional anaesthesia is by using an implanted catheter.[25–29] This may prove to be a useful technique to provide postoperative analgesia for these patients. The effect of engorged orbital contents on the volume of anaesthetic that can be injected may limit the utility of this technique for the subsequent second operation.

References

1   Grossniklaus H, Brown HH, Glasgow BJ, Murray TJ, Sheltar DJ, Wilson DJ, Iserhagen RD. *Ophthalmic pathology and intraocular tumours in basic and clinical science course,* Section 4, 2000–2001. The Foundation of the American Academy of Ophthalmology San Francisco.
2   Scott IU, O'Brien JM, Murray TM. Retinoblastoma: A review emphasizing genetics and management strategies. *Semin Ophthalmol.* 1997; 12:59–71.
3   Murray, TG. Clinical update on retinoblastoma: Current understanding and management. *Fla Ophthalmologist* 1994; 15:8.
4   Scott IU, Moy CS, Murray TG. Update on the collaborative ocular melanoma study (COMS) for the comprehensive ophthalmologist. *Compr Ophthalmol Update.* 2000; 1:185–191.
5   McGoldrick KE. Anatomy and physiology of the eye. In: Zorab R, editor. *Anaesthesia for Ophthalmic and Otolaryngologic Surgery.* Harcourt Brace Jovanovich, Philadelphia, PA, 1992. pp 176–182.
6   Dutton JJ. *Clinical and surgical orbital anatomy.* WB Saunders Company, 1994.
7   The Collaborative Ocular Melanoma Study Group. Mortality in patients with small choroidal melanoma. COMS Report No. 4. *Arch Ophthalmol.* 1997; 115:886–893.
8   Mclean IW, Foster WD, Zimmerman LE. Uveal melanoma: location, size, cell type, and enucleation as risk factors in metastasis. *Hum Pathol.* 1982; 13:123–132.
9   The Collaborative Ocular Melanoma Study Group. Accuracy of diagnosis of choroidal melanomas in the collaborative ocular melanoma study: COMS Report No. 1. *Arch Ophthalmol.* 1990; 108:1268–1273.
10   The Collaborative Ocular Melanoma Study Group. The Collaborative Ocular Melanoma Study randomized trial of pre-enucleation radiation of large choroidal melanoma. I: Characteristics of patients enrolled and not enrolled. COMS Report No. 9. *Am J Ophthalmol.* 1998; 125:767–778.
11   The Collaborative Ocular Melanoma Study Group. The Collaborative Ocular Melanoma Study randomized trial of pre-enucleation radiation of large choroidal melanoma. II: Initial mortality findings. COMS Report No. 10. *Am J Ophthalmol.* 1998; 125:779–796.
12   Augsburger JJ. Is observation really appropriate for small choroidal melanomas? *Trans Am Ophthalmol Soc.* 1993; 91:147–168.
13   The Collaborative Ocular Melanoma Study Group. The Collaborative Ocular Melanoma Study randomized trial of pre-enucleation radiation of large choroidal melanoma. III: Local complications and observations following enucleation. COMS Report No.11. *Am J Ophthalmol.* 1998; 126:362–372.
14   Zimmerman LE, McLean IW, Foster WD. Does enucleation of the eye containing a malignant melanoma prevent or accelerate the dissemination of tumour cells? *Br J Ophthalmol.* 1978; 62:420–425.
15   Ellison N. Problems in geriatric anaesthesia. *Surg Clin North Am.* 1975; 55:929.
16   Stephen CR. The risk of anaesthesia and surgery in the geriatric patient. In: Krechel SW, editor. *Anaesthesia and the geriatric patient.* Grune and Stratton, Orlando, 1984.

17   Munson ES, Hoffman JC, Eger EI. Use of cyclopropane to test generality of anaesthetic requirement in the elderly. *Anesth Analg.* 1984; 63:998.
18   Homer TD, Stanski DR. The effect of increasing age on thiopental disposition and anaesthetic requirement. *Anaesthesiology.* 1985; 62:714–718.
19   McGoldrick, KE. Ophthalmologic and systemic complications of surgery and Anaesthesia. In: *Anaesthesia for ophthalmic and otolaryngologic surgery,* WB Saunders Company, Philadelphia, PA, 1992. pp 278–279.
20   Jedeikin RJ, Hoffman S. The oculocardiac reflex in eye-surgery anaesthesia. *Anesth Analg.* 1977; 56:333.
21   Berler DK. The oculocardiac reflex. *Am J Ophthalmol.* 1963; 12:954–959.
22   Moonie GT, Rees DI, Elton D. Oculocardiac reflex during strabismus surgery. *Can Anaesth Soc J.* 1964; 11:621.
23   van den Berg AA, Lambourne A, Clayburn PA. The oculoemetic reflex, a rationalization of postophthalmic anaesthesia vomiting. *Anaesthesia.* 1989; 44:110–17.
24   The Collaborative Ocular Melanoma Study Group. Complications of enucleation surgery. COMS Report No. 2. In: Franklin RM, editor. *Proceedings of the New Orleans Academy of Ophthalmology Symposium on Retina and Vitreous.* Kugler, The Hague, Netherlands, 1993. pp 181–190.
25   Tamai M. A Retained retrobulbar catheter for repetitive injection of anaesthetics during ophthalmic surgery. *Ophthalmic Surgery* 1983; 14:579–558.
26   Bernard JM, Hommeril JL. Prolonged peribulbar anaesthesia with indwelling catheter: A preliminary report of 217 cases. *Br J Anaesth.* 1997; 78:81–82.
27   Lincoff H, Kreissig I. A catheter to deliver retrobulbar medication. *Arch Ophthalmol.* 1996; 114:634–635.
28   Fezza JP, Klippenstein KA, Wesley RE. Use of an orbital epidural catheter to control pain after orbital implant surgery. *Arch Ophthalmol.* 1999; 117:784–788.
29   Jonas JB, Hemmerling TM, Budde WM, Dinkel M. Postoperative analgesia by re-injections of local anaesthetic through an indwelling retrobulbar catheter. *Am J Ophthalmol.* 2000; 129:54–58.

14

Complications of Ophthalmic Regional Anaesthesia

Dr Robert C. (Roy) Hamilton

Training of the Ophthalmic Regional Anaesthesiologist

Sound knowledge of orbital anatomy, ophthalmic physiology, and the pharmacology of anaesthesia and ophthalmic drugs should be prerequisites before embarking on orbital regional anaesthesia; such information should then be augmented by training in techniques obtained in clinical settings from practitioners with wide experience and knowledge in the field.[1] Clinicians go through an obligatory 'learning curve,' the gradient of which can be reduced by exposure to expert instruction and supervision.[2] To pursue orbital anatomy thoroughly, cadaver dissection is an excellent means of gaining the necessary insights.[3]

Optimal Management of Patients Undergoing Ophthalmic Regional Anaesthesia

All patients require preoperative preparation and assessment with open communication of risks and potential complications that are based on a thorough history and physical examination. This requires cooperation among patients, their family doctors or internists, and surgeon/anaesthetist teams. A list of medications currently taken is required to ensure that essential therapy is continued through the time of surgery and that potential drug interactions can be anticipated. Laboratory and radiological investigations need be ordered only when indicated and appropriate to the management of the case.[4] Ophthalmic surgical patients are often elderly with multiple systemic diseases such as hypertension, coronary artery disease, chronic obstructive pulmonary disease, diabetes, and obesity, conditions presenting additional challenges to the operating team. Every effort should be made to have patients in the best possible condition prior to surgery. Most ophthalmic surgery is not urgent; therefore, the date of surgery can be postponed until the status of each patient is optimal.

High standards of perioperative monitoring must be maintained.[5] For patients who may benefit from preoperative sedation, fine judgment is required to select the correct drug dosage to produce a calm patient who remains alert and cooperative. The advantages of regional anaesthesia can be negated rapidly with excessive use of sedation.[6] A recent multi-centre study confirmed that intravenous anaesthetic agents administered to reduce pain and anxiety are associated with an increased incidence of side effects and adverse medical events.[7] Incomplete regional anaesthesia is best managed with block supplementation. To operate in the presence of obvious block failure is to subject the patient to an unpleasant and stressful experience. The use of intravenous sedation to cover gross block inadequacy is hazardous and inappropriate.

Complications of Ophthalmic Regional Anaesthesia

Haemorrhage

Retrobulbar haemorrhages vary in severity. Some are of venous origin and spread slowly. Signs of severe arterial haemorrhage are a rapid and taut orbital swelling, marked proptosis with immobility of the globe, and massive blood staining of the lids and conjunctiva.[8] Serious impairment of the vascular supply to the globe may result.[9] Constant vigilance and keen observation of the signs immediately following needle withdrawal are vital. Bleeding may be minimized and confined by rapid application of digital pressure over a gauze pad applied to the closed lids. The incidence of serious retrobulbar bleeding is reported as high as 3%[10] and 0.44% in a more recent series of 12,500 cases.[11] Gentle and smooth needle insertion without pivotal or slicing movement is less likely to cause bleeding.[10,11] A strong argument can be made in favour of fine disposable needles over those of larger gauge[12–14] on the grounds that if a vessel is perforated, then the amount of bleeding that occurs through a small rent is of lesser amount and less precipitous.

The anterior orbit has smaller vessels than exist posteriorly. In the interest of avoiding haemorrhage, sites that are relatively avascular are preferable for needle placement. The inferotemporal quadrant and the medial canthal periconal compartment are recommended. The superonasal quadrant of the orbit should be avoided because the end vessels of the ophthalmic artery are located there, as is the complex trochlear mechanism of the superior oblique muscle. Since orbital blood vessels are largest in the posterior orbit, deep needle placement must be avoided (see next section).

Brainstem Anaesthesia

Brainstem anaesthesia may occur with ophthalmic regional anaesthesia.[15] It is not caused by increasing levels of drug in the systemic circulation (including CNS) but by direct spread of local anaesthetic to the brain from the orbit along sub-meningeal pathways. Clinical doses of local anaesthetics used in eye surgery do not result usually in high and dangerous systemic levels. Brainstem anaesthesia, which the literature reports as occurring with an incidence of 1 in 350 to 500 intraconal local anaesthesia injections,[15] may require cardiopulmonary resuscitation. Typically the patient first describes symptoms with onset at about 2 minutes after the orbital injection but these may be delayed for 10 to 20 minutes, resolving over 2 to 3 hours. As this is a potential complication on each occasion that orbital blocks are performed, patients should not be draped for surgery until 15 minutes have elapsed after completion of the block, otherwise identification and corrective treatment may be delayed dangerously. The provision of pulse oximetry in the block room and operating room[13] is an essential prerequisite in all locations where regional ocular anaesthesia is performed. Equipment to provide respiratory support and cardiopulmonary resuscitation[8,16–19] must also be readily available. The clinical picture of brainstem anaesthesia is unpredictable. Signs may vary from mild confusion, through marked shivering or fitting, bilateral cranial nerve palsies (including motor nerve blocking to the contralateral orbit with amaurosis) or hemi-, para-, or quadriplegia, with or without loss of consciousness, to apnoea with marked cardiovascular instability.[15] Central spread should be suspected if any of these signs is observed.

Treatment of these differing manifestations of central spread includes reassurance, ventilatory support with oxygen, intravenous fluid therapy, and pharmacological circulatory support with vagolytics, vasopressors, vasodilators or adrenergic blocking agents as appropriate and as dictated by close vital sign monitoring.

Much is known about prevention of this syndrome. Unsöld and co-workers in 1981[20] exposed the danger of the elevated, adducted globe, as advocated by Atkinson,[21] during inferotemporal needle placement. This position places the optic nerve closer to the advancing needle. They demonstrated in computed tomography studies in the fresh cadaver that with the globe in primary gaze the optic nerve is less vulnerable. Avoidance of deep penetration of the orbit in any technique is advisable both to prevent this and other serious block complications. Katsev et al. advised that maximum penetration from the orbit rim should be 31 mm.[22] Modern techniques advocate more shallow injections relying on larger volumes of injectate to spread to the apex.

Globe Penetration and Perforation

The perception of changes in tissue densities during needle advancement is a vital part of safe regional anaesthesia; it is an acquired skill that requires experience and ongoing practice.[23] Needle advancement within the confines of the orbit is a blind procedure and has the potential of serious complications. Although the complication rate is low, because of the large numbers of eye block procedures carried out annually, even rare complications become significant.[24] The Atkinson 'up and in' globe positioning[21] has been discredited. During inferotemporal needle insertion with the globe elevated and adducted, the optic nerve is brought closer to the needle tip and the macular area is more exposed to damage.[18,20,22,25] Optic nerve sheath penetration, optic nerve trauma and ocular penetration or perforation by the needle may result. The posterior pole of the globe is endangered, particularly in the ovoid globes of myopic patients.[12] Many serious complications are avoided by having patients direct their eyes in primary gaze position during needle placement and subsequent injection. In the literature there was a considerable lobby for the use of dull needles to reduce the incidence of bleeding and of ocular penetration.[26–28] No controlled trial has demonstrated any superiority of blunt over sharp-tipped needles in reducing these complications.[29] Grizzard states that tactile discrimination is progressively reduced with increasing needle size. The increased resistance caused by a blunt needle is not appreciated because of the necessarily greater force required for insertion.[12] Grizzard et al., reporting on iatrogenic ocular injuries, found that penetration or perforation of the eye from use of larger dull needles caused more serious damage than when fine disposable ones were implicated and questioned the arguments in the earlier literature that advocated their use.[30] This was the first report in the literature showing an advantage of sharp over blunt needles other than patient comfort. Using blunt-tipped needles does not convey protection against penetration; of the twenty-three cases reported by Hay et al., seven were caused by dull needles and of the eleven reported by Grizzard et al., five implicated this type of needle.[30,31] Because the ratio of resistances of scleral to skin penetration remained the same for needle tips of both the sharp and dull varieties, Vivian and Canning concluded that it was unlikely that dull needles offered any protection against the complication.[24] Blunt-tipped needles are painful for the patient, whereas fine disposable needles cause much less discomfort and with their use oral and intravenous sedative medication often become unnecessary. The use of blunt-tipped, wider-gauge needles should be abandoned.[32]

Although there are proponents of both intraconal and periconal techniques, safe anaesthesia can be accomplished by both methods; likewise, serious complications can arise with both if carried out incorrectly. A faster onset of anaesthesia is achieved when blocking within the muscle cone.[13,33] Approximately 10% of peribublar blocks are considered failures because they do not provide adequate ocular analgesia.[34] Chemosis is more common with periconal blocks.[35] Whilst it is possible to get superb blocks with small volume injection at the apex of the orbit,[36] the risks are too great. 31 mm as measured from the orbit rim should never be exceeded[22] nor should a needle advancing from an inferotemporal entry be allowed to cross the mid-sagittal plane of the eye (Figure 1).[12]

All needles used for intraconal and periconal insertion should be orientated tangentially to the globe with the bevel opening faced toward the globe.[13,37] If a tangentially aligned needle contacts the sclera, globe penetration is less likely to occur than with a needle approaching at a greater angle. All needles in the orbit are potentially hazardous in the wrong hands; careful supervision and training in technique have great relevance in the avoidance of serious complications.[1] Techniques requiring multiple needle placements are associated with an increased incidence of complications when compared with a single or reduced number of injections.

To avoid scleral penetration (entrance wound only) or perforation (entrance and exit wounds) the importance of block technique and needle type are stressed. The equator of the globe, with the eye in the primary position, is the greatest diameter in the coronal plane. Any needle entering the orbital region anteriorly must be directed in such a manner as to avoid encountering the sclera. Only by accurately judging the position of the equator can a needle be inserted in safety.[1] The author, with an

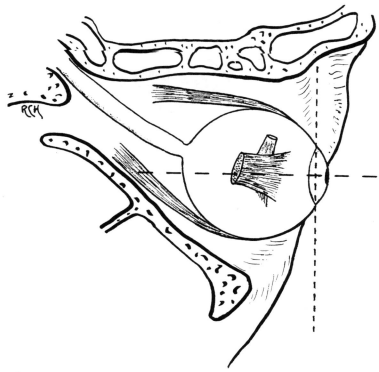

Fig. 1. View from above. Globe in primary gaze. Fine dashed line indicates the plane of the iris; coarse dashed line indicates the mid-sagittal plane of the eye and the visual axis through the centre of the pupil and the retinal macula. The optic nerve lies on the nasal side of the mid-sagittal plane of the eye. Note how the temporal orbit rim is set back from the rest of the orbit rim at or about the globe equator, making for easy needle access to the retrobulbar compartment. (From Gimbel Educational Services, with permission.)

experience of over 33,000 retrobulbar (intraconal) blocks, routinely uses and recommends a percutaneous approach from a more lateral inferotemporal entry point than commonly practised,[38] after preliminary local anaesthesia of the skin (Figure 2).[39] By using a percutaneous entry, patients with narrow palpebral fissures and strongly blinking patients present no problem.

Ocular penetration or perforation is more likely in patients with elongated myopic eyes. Patients presenting for retinal detachment or refractive surgery (such as radial keratotomy and photorefractive keratectomy) have a higher likelihood of longer globes than patients having cataract surgery. Reported incidence of globe penetration and perforation in the literature ranges from none in a series of 2,000 periconal blocks,[40] through one in a series of 12,000 comprising both peri- and intraconal,[13] one in a series of 1000,[41] to three in a series of 4,000 intraconal blocks.[42] Duker et al. state that in myopic patients the incidence may be as high as 1 in 140.[43] There are case reports of the complication with both the intraconal and the periconal methods. Non-akinetic anaesthesia methods have been developed (see below), partly to avoid

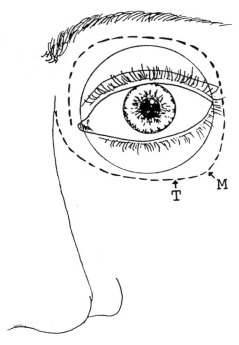

Fig. 2.   The outline of the globe is superimposed on a template of the orbit rim. The traditional inferior
block injection site ('T') is just inside the orbit rim at the junction of the medial two-thirds and
lateral third of the inferior orbital rim. The author's modified injection site ('M') is just inside
the orbit rim at the junction of the inferior and lateral orbital rims. Injection at the modified site
is best done percutaneously, the entry point on the skin being 4 to 5 mm inferior to the lateral
canthus. (From Gimbel Educational Services, with permission.)

the serious complications, including scleral penetration/perforation, related to full
akinetic ophthalmic regional anaesthesia. A prerequisite to regional anaesthesia of
the orbit is to know the axial length measurement of the eye prior to the block to
warn of the higher risk in long eyes. In cataract surgery a precise axial length measurement is usually available as it is required for intraocular lens dioptre power calculation. In other procedures where the axial length is not precisely known, close
attention to the dioptre power of patients' spectacles or contact lenses will provide
valuable clues to globe dimensions. Fine disposable needles, which are less painful
for the patient, have been proven to be relatively safe; however, excellent knowledge
of orbital anatomy is essential. The diagnosis of penetration may be suspected in the
presence of hypotony, poor red reflex, vitreous haemorrhage, and 'a poking through
sensation;'[44] however, more than 50% of needle penetrations of the globe go
unrecognised at the time of their occurrence.[45] The patient may report marked pain
at the time of the penetration,[46] particularly if the anaesthetic is injected intraocu-
larly. Fundoscopy confirms the diagnosis if the media are sufficiently clear. Cases
involving retinal tears only, with minimal bloodstaining of the vitreous, can be managed with laser photocoagulation, cryotherapy, or on occasion observation only.

When so much blood is present that the fundus is not visible, early vitrectomy may be indicated. Without surgical intervention vitreous haemorrhage following penetrating injury frequently leads to proliferative vitreoretinopathy with resultant detachment of the retina. Once retinal detachment is diagnosed, whether associated with clear or cloudy media, prompt surgical treatment is indicated. The appropriate management of scleral penetration and perforation is complex and often drawn out over some weeks involving difficult judgement calls on the part of the ophthalmologist.[47]

The occurrence of ocular explosion associated with orbital blockade, a devastating complication with catastrophic visual outcome, has been described.[48,49] It occurs following unrecognised ocular penetration followed by use of excessive force of local anaesthetic injection. To date eight cases have been described in the literature. The precautions described above, if adequately studied, understood and followed, should make this complication impossible.

Myotoxicity

Prolonged extraocular muscle malfunction may follow regional anaesthesia of the orbit.[13,50,51] Diplopia and ptosis are common for 24 to 48 hours postoperatively when long-acting local anaesthetics have been used in large volume; however, when this persists for days or weeks, or fails to recover, it may be evidence of toxic change within muscle. If muscle recovery is delayed more than six weeks, 25% of the patients will have permanent dysfunction. It is indeed a complication of the greatest magnitude for a patient to have an excellent optical result and end up with devastating diplopia. Studies of the myotoxicity of local anaesthetics have been published.[52–54] Higher concentrations of local anaesthetic agents are more likely to result in myotoxicity.[54] A common cause of prolonged muscle malfunction, whatever concentration has been used, is intramuscular injection.[52,53,55,56] The aetiologies of these muscle malfunctions, however, include not only local anaesthetic myotoxicity,[52–54] but also surgical trauma, inappropriately placed antibiotic injection[57] and ischaemic contracture of the Volkmann's type following trauma/haemorrhage.[58] Increasing age is associated with poor recovery from anaesthesia-induced muscle damage.[59] It is imperative to have a good three-dimensional knowledge of the anatomy of the orbit and its contents to accurately place injections. Of particular note are the number of articles indicating damage to the inferior rectus muscle,[56,60–63] most likely caused by inadequate elevation of the needle tip from the orbit floor during attempted intraconal placement (Figure 3).

By meticulous attention to the placement of anaesthetic needles and with precise knowledge of the anatomy of the six extraocular muscles, the incidence of muscle damage/malfunction can be minimised. Hamed's article in February 1991[58] stressed the importance of aiming the retrobulbar needle 'midway between the inferior and lateral rectus muscles' to gain clear entry into the intraconal space, avoiding trauma to the inferior rectus muscle. There was a suggestion in the paper to move the entry point of the retrobulbar injection to the temporal side. Extraocular muscles are more easily avoided by using a fully inferotemporal orbital entry point for the retrobulbar

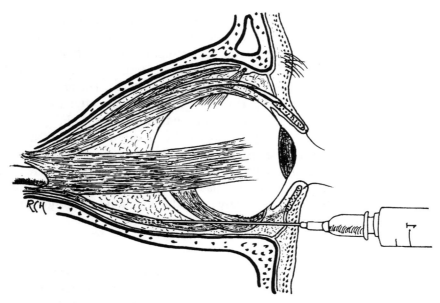

Fig. 3. A straight 31 mm needle being advanced from the inferotemporal quadrant in an attempt to
enter the intraconal space has failed to adequately clear the orbit floor. The needle tip has
entered the belly of the inferior rectus muscle. Haemorrhage into the muscle with subsequent
fibrosis, or intramuscular injection of local anaesthetic with subsequent myotoxicity, may result
in prolonged or permanent imbalance between the superior and inferior rectus muscles and vertical diplopia. (From Gimbel Educational Services, with permission.)

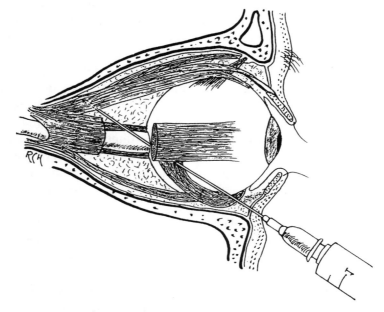

Fig. 4. A straight 38 mm (1½") needle being advanced from the inferotemporal quadrant has traversed
the intracone space and entered the belly of the superior rectus muscle. (From Gimbel Educational Services, with permission.)

injection (Figure 2).[38] This entry point for the retrobulbar block provides safer access to the intraconal space, since the orbit rim is most posterior temporally (Figure 1). Vertical strabismus may be due to superior rectus damage; the tip of a 38mm (1½") retrobulbar needle may enter the superior rectus from an inferotemporal approach (Figure 4),[64] or a bridle traction suture may be responsible.[65] Inferior oblique muscle injury and trauma to its motor nerve by regional anaesthesia injection have been reported.[59] Less commonly affected are the superior oblique,[66] the medial rectus (Figure 5)[67], and the lateral rectus.[68] Persistent strabismus may be caused by contracture of an antagonist muscle reacting to an initial temporary paresis of its agonist muscle.[62]

Globe Ischaemia

In intraocular surgery it is considered advantageous if the intraocular pressure is low and pressure fluctuations are kept to a minimum.[69] The attainment of a 'soft eye' in the avoidance of complications, particularly suprachoroidal haemorrhage,[70] was more important in a former era. Phacoemulsification techniques, which require a smaller surgical incision, are associated with smaller swings in intraocular pressure than the older intracapsular or extracapsular methods. Following completion of regional anaesthetic blocks mechanical orbital decompression devices[71-74] are commonly used to promote ocular hypotony and reduced vitreous volume,[75] especially when larger volumes of orbital injectate have been used (as in periconal blocks).

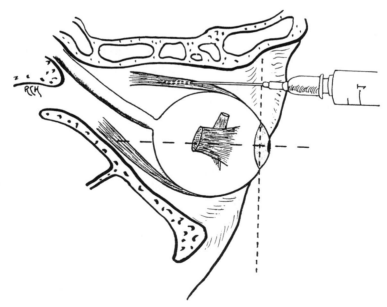

Fig. 5. A straight needle being advanced in a sagittal plane from the extreme medial end of the palpebral fissure (on the nasal side of the caruncle) has traversed the medial compartment on the nasal side of the medial rectus muscle and entered into the belly of the medial rectus muscle. (From Gimbel Educational Services, with permission.)

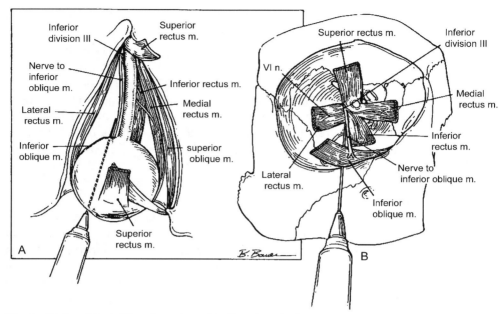

Fig. 6.   Right orbit: A. View from above. B. View from in front with the globe removed. Observe the proximity of the needle path to the inferior oblique muscle belly, its motor nerve and the lateral border of the inferior rectus muscle. One or more of these three structures can be damaged by a traditionally placed retrobulbar needle. (From Hunter et al.,[59] with permission.)

Since blood flow to the retina, choroid and optic nerve depends on the balance between the intraocular pressure and the mean local arterial blood pressure, it is possible for these devices to induce globe ischaemia.[76,77] In the presence of significant local arterial disease, orbital haemorrhage or in patients with glaucoma, vascular occlusion may result.[78] It may be prudent to omit epinephrine from the anaesthesia injectate in these cases.[12,33]

Optic Nerve Damage

Injection at the orbital apex has the potential of frank optic nerve injury. It is possible for the needle tip to enter the optic nerve sheath and produce not only brainstem anaesthesia but also tamponade of the retinal vessels within the nerve and/or the small vessels supplying the nerve itself either by the volume of drug injected or by causing intrasheath haemorrhage.[10,14,79–81] Even without trauma to the optic nerve the increased orbital pressure of retrobulbar haemorrhage may tamponade its small nutrient vessels, which may explain those cases of profound visual loss in which the findings of retinal vascular occlusion were not seen and late optic atrophy developed.[8,78] Pre-existing small vessel disease may increase the likelihood of this complication.

Other Nerve Injury

It is possible for any of the nerves[59,82,83] in the orbit to be traumatized by a needle. The nerve to the inferior oblique muscle may be damaged by a needle advancing along the orbit floor (Figure 6) with resultant diplopia,[59] if this is not inserted sufficiently lateral.

Therapeutic Misadventures

Orbital injections of depot steroid medications and antibiotics are frequently employed at the time of ophthalmic surgery for their anti-inflammatory and anti-infective properties. Their inadvertent injection into the vitreous has serious implications.[84–90] In delivering steroids and antibiotics in a planned extraocular location, it is important to aspirate prior to injection to check for inadvertent intravascular needle-tip placement. There are reports of retinal, ciliary and choroidal arterial embolism of these medications, often with irreversible visual deterioration.[91–93]

The incidence of systemic toxicity with local anaesthetics is related to total dose given, vascularity of site of injection, drug used, speed of injection, and whether epinephrine has been used as an additive to delay systemic release. The amount of local anaesthesia agent required to be effective in ophthalmologic practice is relatively small, so systemic toxicity is less likely. Aspirating before injection and injecting slowly reduce the likelihood of this complication. Inadvertent intra-arterial injection of local anaesthetics with retrograde flow to the cerebral circulation may result in an acute grand mal seizure.[94,95]

Seventh Nerve Block Complications

An isolated facial nerve block is rarely necessary in modern ophthalmic practice. Complications of blocking the main trunk of the facial nerve at the base of the skull have been reported.[96,97] These include difficulty in swallowing and breathing related to unilateral vagus, glossopharyngeal, phrenic and spinal accessory blockade. For facial nerve blockade below the ear, injections should not be deeper than 12 mm and hyaluronidase should be avoided.[97,98] Bilateral block must never be done.[99]

Allergy

True allergy to local anaesthetics is extremely rare.[100] Allergic reactions are almost exclusively confined to the ester-linked drugs. The breakdown product para-aminobenzoic acid (PABA) of the esters is thought to trigger the allergic reaction in certain individuals. Crossreaction with preservatives, such as methylparabens, in multidose vials is possible, and it may be better to use preservative-free vials where a history of the problem exists.[101] Patients have been reported who exhibit a myasthenia-like response to various agents including local anaesthetics[102] and two well-documented cases of true allergy to amide drugs have been reported in the literature.[103,104]

Anticoagulants and Antiplatelet Therapy

Reducing or discontinuing anticoagulant therapy for some days prior to surgery has been a common practice. This may be appropriate for major ophthalmic surgical procedures, such as scleral buckling, but the balance of risk for cataract surgery favours its continuation.[105,106] Stopping anticoagulants may result in thrombotic complications such as cerebral vascular accident, pulmonary embolism, and death.[107] The minor haemorrhagic complications associated with maintaining anticoagulation have had no long-term effects on visual acuity.[108,109] Patients on antiplatelet therapy may also continue their drugs through cataract surgery if medically indicated.[110]

References

1   Hawkesworth NR. Peribulbar anaesthesia [letter]. *Br J Ophthalmol.* 1992; 76:254.
2   Kopacz DJ, Neal JM, Pollock MD. The regional anesthesia 'learning curve'. What is the minimum number of epidural and spinal blocks to reach consistency? *Reg Anesth.* 1996; 21:182–190.
3   Wong DHW. Regional anaesthesia for intraocular surgery [review]. *Can J Anaesth.* 1993; 40:635–657.
4   Schein OD, Katz J, Bass E, Tielsch JM, Lubomski LH, Feldman MA, Petty BG, Steinberg EP. The value of routine preoperative medical testing before cataract surgery: a randomized trial. *N Engl J Med.* 2000; 342:168–175.
5   Rubin AP. Anaesthesia for cataract surgery — time for change? [editorial]. *Anaesthesia.* 1990; 45:717–718.
6   Smith DC, Crul JF. Oxygen desaturation following sedation for regional analgesia. *Br J Anaesth.* 1989; 62:206–209.
7   Katz J, Feldman MA, Bass EB, Lubomski LH, Tielsch JM, Petty BG, Fleisher LA, Schein OD. Adverse intraoperative medical events and their association with anesthesia management strategies in cataract surgery. *Ophthalmology.* 2001; 108:1721–1726.
8   Feibel RM. Current concepts in retrobulbar anesthesia. *Surv Ophthalmol.* 1985; 30:102–110.
9   Puustjarvi T, Purhonen S. Permanent blindness following retrobulbar hemorrhage after peribulbar anesthesia for cataract surgery. *Ophthalmic Surg.* 1992; 23:450–452.
10   Morgan CM, Schatz H, Vine AK, Cantril HL, Davidorf FH, Gitter KA, Rudich R. Ocular complications associated with retrobulbar injections. *Ophthalmology.* 1988; 95:660–665.
11   Edge KR, Nicoll JMV. Retrobulbar hemorrhage after 12,500 retrobulbar blocks. *Anesth Analg.* 1993; 76:1019–1022.
12   Grizzard WS. Ophthalmic anesthesia. In: Reinecke RD, editor. *Ophthalmology Annual.* New York: Raven Press, 1989; 265–294.
13   Hamilton RC, Gimbel HV, Strunin L. Regional anaesthesia for 12,000 cataract extraction and intraocular lens implantation procedures. *Can J Anaesth.* 1988; 35:615–623.
14   Pautler SE, Grizzard WS, Thompson LN, Wing GL. Blindness from retrobulbar injection into the optic nerve. *Ophthalmic Surg.* 1986; 17:334–337.
15   Hamilton RC. Brain-stem anesthesia as a complication of regional anesthesia for ophthalmic surgery. *Can J Ophthalmol.* 1992; 27:323–325.
16   Fletcher SJ, O'Sullivan G. Grand mal seizure after retrobulbar block. *Anaesthesia.* 1990; 45:696.
17   Hamilton RC. Brain stem anesthesia following retrobulbar blockade. *Anesthesiology.* 1985; 63:688–690.

18   Javitt JC, Addiego R, Friedberg HL, Libonati MM, Leahy JJ. Brain stem anesthesia after retrobulbar block. *Ophthalmology.* 1987; 94:718–724.
19   Morgan GE. Retrobulbar apnea syndrome: A case for the routine presence of an anesthesiologist [letter]. *Reg Anesth.* 1990; 15:106–107.
20   Unsöld R, Stanley JA, DeGroot J. The CT-topography of retrobulbar anesthesia. *A Graef Arch Klin Exp Ophthalmol.* 1981; 217:125–136.
21   Atkinson WS. Retrobulbar injection of anesthetic within the muscular cone (cone injection). *Arch Ophthalmol.* 1936; 16:494–503.
22   Katsev DA, Drews RC, Rose BT. An anatomic study of retrobulbar needle path length. *Ophthalmology.* 1989; 96:1221–1224.
23   Brown DL, Wedel DJ. Introduction to regional anesthesia. In: Miller RD, editor. *Anesthesia.* 3rd ed. New York: Churchill Livingstone, 1990; 1369–1375.
24   Vivian AJ, Canning CR. Scleral perforation with retrobulbar needles. *Eur J Implant Ref Surg.* 1993; 5:39–41.
25   Liu C, Youl B, Moseley I. Magnetic resonance imaging of the optic nerve in extremes of gaze. Implications for the positioning of the globe for retrobulbar anaesthesia. *Br J Ophthalmol.* 1992; 76:728–733.
26   Callahan A. Ultrasharp disposable needles [letter]. *Am J Ophthalmol.* 1966; 62:173.
27   Davis DB, Mandel MR. Posterior peribulbar anesthesia: An alternative to retrobulbar anesthesia. *J Cataract Refract Surg.* 1986; 12:182–184.
28   Kimble JA, Morris RE, Witherspoon CD, Feist RM. Globe perforation from peribulbar injection. *Arch Ophthalmol.* 1987; 105:749.
29   Dhaliwal R, Demediuk OM. A comparison of peribulbar and retrobulbar anesthesia for vitreoretinal surgical procedures [comment]. *Arch Ophthalmol.* 1996; 114:502.
30   Grizzard WS, Kirk NM, Pavan PR, Antworth MV, Hammer ME, Roseman RL. Perforating ocular injuries caused by anesthesia personnel. *Ophthalmology.* 1991; 98:1011–1016.
31   Hay A, Flynn HWJr, Hoffman JI, Rivera AH. Needle penetration of the globe during retrobulbar and peribulbar injections. *Ophthalmology.* 1991; 98:1017–1024.
32   Gardner S, Ryall D. Local anaesthesia within the orbit. *Curr Anaesth Crit Care.* 2000; 11:299–305.
33   Loots JH, Koorts AS, Venter JA. Peribulbar anesthesia. A prospective statistical analysis of the efficacy and predictability of bupivacaine and a lignocaine/bupivacaine mixture. *J Cataract Refract Surg.* 1993; 19:72–76.
34   McGoldrick KE. *Anesthesia for Ophthalmic and Otolaryngologic Surgery.* Saunders, Philadelphia, 1992. pp 272–290.
35   Weiss JL, Deichman CB. A comparison of retrobulbar and periocular anesthesia for cataract surgery. *Arch Ophthalmol.* 1989; 107:96–98.
36   Gifford H. Motor block of extraocular muscles by deep orbital injection. *Arch Ophthalmol.* 1949; 41:5–19.
37   Gills JP, Loyd TL. A technique of retrobulbar block with paralysis of orbicularis oculi. *J Am Intraocular Implant Soc.* 1983; 9:339–340.
38   Hamilton RC. Retrobulbar block revisited and revised. *J Cataract Refract Surg.* 1996; 22:1147–1150.
39   Hamilton RC. Retrobulbar anesthesia. *Oper Tech Cataract Refract Surg.* 2000; 3:116–121.
40   Davis DB, Mandel MR. Posterior peribulbar anesthesia: An alternative to retrobulbar anesthesia. *J Cataract Refract Surg.* 1986; 12:182–184.
41   Cibis PA. Discussion. In: Schepens CL, Regan CDJ, editors. *Controversial Aspects of the Management of Retinal Detactments.* Little, Brown, Boston, 1965. p 251.
42   Ramsay RC, Knobloch WH. Ocular perforation following retrobulbar anesthesia for retinal detachment surgery. *Am J Ophthalmol.* 1978; 86:61–64.

43   Duker JS, Belmont JB, Benson WE, Brooks HL, Brown GC, Federman JL, Fischer DH, Tasman WS. Inadvertent globe perforation during retrobulbar and peribulbar anesthesia. *Ophthalmology.* 1991; 98:519–526.

44   Gentili ME, Brassier J. Is peribulbar block safer than retrobulbar? [letter] *Reg Anesth.* 1992; 17:309.

45   Ginsburg RN, Duker JS. Globe perforation associated with retrobulbar and peribulbar anesthesia. *Sem Ophthalmol.* 1993; 8:87–95.

46   Seelenfreund MH, Freilich DB. Retinal injuries associated with cataract surgery. *Am J Ophthalmol.* 1980; 89:654–658.

47   Rinkoff JS, Doft BH, Lobes LA. Management of ocular penetration from injection of local anesthesia preceding cataract surgery. *Arch Ophthalmol.* 1991; 109:1421–1425.

48   Magnante DO, Bullock JD, Green WR. Ocular explosion after peribulbar anesthesia: case report and experimental study. *Ophthalmology.* 1997; 104:608–615.

49   Bullock JD, Warwar RE, Green WR. Ocular explosions from periocular anesthetic injections. A clinical, histopathologic, experimental, and biophysical study. *Ophthalmology.* 1999; 106:2341–2353.

50   Carlson BM, Emerick S, Komorowski TE, Rainin EA, Shepard BM. Extraocular muscle regeneration in primates. *Ophthalmology.* 1992; 99:582–589.

51   Rao VA, Kawatra VK. Ocular myotoxic effects of local anesthetics. *Can J Ophthalmol.* 1988; 23:171–173.

52   Foster AH, Carlson BM. Myotoxicity of local anesthetics and regeneration of the damaged muscle fibers. *Anesth Analg.* 1980; 59:727–736.

53   Rainin EA, Carlson BM. Postoperative diplopia and ptosis; a clinical hypothesis on the myotoxicity of local anesthetics. *Arch Ophthalmol.* 1985; 103:1337–1339.

54   Yagiela JA, Benoit PW, Buoncristiani RD, Peters MP, Fort NF. Comparison of myotoxic effects of lidocaine with epinephrine in rats and humans. *Anesth Analg.* 1981; 60:471–480.

55   O'Brien CS. Local anesthesia. *Arch Ophthalmol.* 1934; 12:240–253.

56   Ong-Tone L, Pearce WG. Inferior rectus muscle restriction after retrobulbar anesthesia for cataract extraction. *Can J Ophthalmol.* 1989; 24:162–165.

57   Kushner BJ. Ocular muscle fibrosis following cataract extraction. *Arch Ophthalmol.* 1988; 106:18–19.

58   Hamed LM. Strabismus presenting after cataract surgery. *Ophthalmology.* 1991; 98:247–252.

59   Hunter DG, Lam GC, Guyton DL. Inferior oblique muscle injury from local anesthesia for cataract surgery. *Ophthalmology.* 1995; 102:501–509.

60   Burns CL, Seigel LA. Inferior rectus recession for vertical tropia after cataract surgery. *Ophthalmology.* 1988; 95:1120–1124.

61   de Faber J-THN, von Noorden GK. Inferior rectus muscle palsy after retrobulbar anesthesia for cataract surgery [letter]. *Am J Ophthalmol.* 1991; 112:209–211.

62   Grimmett MR, Lambert SR. Superior rectus muscle overaction after cataract extraction. *Am J Ophthalmol.* 1992; 114:72–80.

63   Hamed LM, Mancuso A. Inferior rectus muscle contracture syndrome after retrobulbar anesthesia. *Ophthalmology.* 1991; 98:1506–1512.

64   Capó H, Roth E, Johnson T, Munoz M, Siatkowski RM. Vertical strabismus after cataract surgery. *Ophthalmology.* 1996; 103:918–921.

65   Catalano RA, Nelson LB, Caljoun JH, Schatz NJ. Harley RD. Persistent strabismus presenting after cataract surgery. *Ophthalmology.* 1987; 94:491–494.

66   Erie JC. Acquired Brown's syndrome after peribulbar anesthesia. *Am J Ophthalmol.* 1990; 109:349–350.

67   Hustead RF, Hamilton RC, Loken RG. Periocular local anesthesia: medial orbital as an alternative to superior nasal injection. *J Cataract Refract Surg.* 1994; 20:197–201.

68 Barrere M. Cut risk of strabismus. *Ophthalmol Times.* 1995; March 27–April 2:12.
69 Mackool RJ. Intraocular pressure fluctuations [letter]. *J Cataract Refract Surg.* 1993; 19:563–564.
70 Atkinson WS. Observations on anesthesia for ocular surgery. *Trans Am Acad Ophthalmol Otolaryngol.* 1956; 60:376–380.
71 Buys NS. Mercury balloon reducer for vitreous and orbital volume control. In: Emery J, editor. *Current Concepts in Cataract Surgery.* CV Mosby, St. Louis, 1980. p 258.
72 Davidson B, Kratz R, Mazzoco T. An evaluation of the Honan intraocular pressure reducer. *J Am Intraocular Implant Soc.* 1979; 5:237–238.
73 Drews RC. The Nerf ball for preoperative reduction of introcular pressure. *Ophthalmic Surgery* 1982; 13:761.
74 Gills JP. Constant mild compression of the eye to produce hypotension. *J Am Intraocular Implant Soc.* 1979; 5:52–53.
75 Palay DA, Stulting RD. The effect of external ocular compression on intraocular pressure following retrobulbar anesthesia. *Ophthalmic Surgery* 1990; 21:503–507.
76 Jay WM, Aziz MZ, Green K. Effect of Honan intraocular pressure reducer on ocular and optic nerve blood flow in phakic rabbit eyes. *Acta Ophthalmol.* 1986; 64:52–57.
77 Loken RG, Coupland SG, Deschênes MC. The electroretinogram during orbital compression following intraorbital (regional) block for cataract surgery. *Can J Anaesth.* 1994; 41:802–806.
78 Carl JR. Optic neuropathy following cataract extraction. *Semin Ophthalmol.* 1993; 8:144–148.
79 Brod RD. Transient central retinal occlusion and contralateral amaurosis after retrobulbar anesthetic injection. *Ophthalmic Surgery* 1989; 20:643–646.
80 Giuffrè G, Vadala M, Manfrè L. Retrobulbar anesthesia complicated by combined central retinal vein and artery occlusion and massive vitreoretinal fibrosis. *Retina.* 1995; 15:439–441.
81 Sullivan KL, Brown GC, Forman AR, Sergott RC, Flanagan JC. Retrobulbar anesthesia and retinal vascular obstruction. *Ophthalmology.* 1983; 90:373–377.
82 Lam S, Beck RW, Hall D, Creighton JB. Atonic pupil after cataract surgery. *Ophthalmology.* 1989; 96:589–590.
83 Saiz A, Angulo S, Fernandez M. Atonic pupil: An unusual complication of cataract surgery. *Ophthalmic Surgery* 1991; 22:20–22.
84 Brown GC, Eagle RC, Shakin EP, Gruber M, Arbizion VV. Retinal toxicity of intravitreal gentamicin. *Arch Ophthalmol.* 1990; 108:1740–1744.
85 Campochiaro PA, Conway BP. Aminoglycoside toxicity – a survey of retinal specialists: implications for ocular use. *Arch Ophthalmol.* 1991; 109:946–950.
86 Jain VK, Mames RN, McGorray S, Giles CL. Inadvertent penetrating injury to the globe with periocular corticosteroid injection. *Ophthalmic Surgery* 1991; 22:508–511.
87 Nianiaris NA, Mandelcorn M, Baker G. Retinal and choroidal embolization following soft-tissue maxillary injection of corticosteroids. *Can J Ophthalmol.* 1995; 30:321–323.
88 Pendergast SD, Eliott D, Machemer R. Retinal toxic effects following inadvertent intraocular injection of Celestone Soluspan [letter]. *Arch Ophthalmol.* 1995; 113:1230–1231.
89 Schlaegal TF, Wilson FM. Accidental intraocular injection of depot corticosteroids. *Trans Am Acad Ophthalmol Otolaryngol.* 1974; 78:847–855.
90 Verma LK, Goyal M, Tewari HK. Inadvertent intraocular injection of depot corticosteroids. *Ophthalmic Surg Laser.* 1996; 27:73–74.
91 Ellis PP. Occlusion of the central retinal artery after retrobulbar corticosteroid injection. *Am J Ophthalmol.* 1978; 85:352–356.

92   McLean EB. Inadvertent injection of corticosteroid into the choroidal vasculature. *Am J Ophthalmol.* 1975; 80:835–837.

93   Shorr N, Seiff SR. Central retinal artery occlusion associated with periocular corticosteroid injection for juvenile hemangioma. *Ophthalmic Surgery* 1986; 17:229–231.

94   Aldrete JA, Romo-Salas F, Arora S, Wilson R, Rutherford R. Reverse arterial blood flow as a pathway for central nervous system toxic responses following injection of local anesthetics. *Anesth Analg.* 1978; 57:428–433.

95   Meyers EF, Ramirez RC, Boniuk I. Grand mal seizures after retrobulbar block. *Arch Ophthalmol.* 1978; 96:847.

96   Koenig SB, Snyder RW, Kay J. Respiratory distress after a Nadbath block. *Ophthalmology.* 1988; 95:1285–1287.

97   Lindquist TD, Kopietz LA, Spigelman AV, Nichols BD, Lindstrom RL. Complications of Nadbath facial nerve block and review of the literature. *Ophthalmic Surgery* 1988; 19:271–273.

98   Nadbath RP, Rehman I. Facial nerve block. *Am J Ophthalmol.* 1963; 55:143–146.

99   Rabinowitz L, Livingston M, Schneider H, Hall A. Respiratory obstruction following the Nadbath facial nerve block [letter]. *Arch Ophthalmol.* 1986; 104:1115.

100 Philip BK, Covino BG. Local and regional anesthesia. In: Wetchler BV, editor. *Anesthesia for Ambulatory Surgery.* 2nd ed. JB Lippincott Company, Philadelphia, 1991. p 357.

101 Incaudo G, Schatz M, Patterson R, Rosenberg M, Yamamoto F, Hamburger RN. Administration of local anesthetics to patients with a history of prior adverse reaction. *J Allergy Clin Immunol.* 1978; 61:339–345.

102 Meyer D, Hamilton RC, Gimbel HV. Myasthenia gravis-like syndrome induced by topical ophthalmic preparations. A case report. *J Clin Neuroophthalmol.* 1992; 12:210–212.

103 Brown DT, Beamish D, Wildsmith JAW. Allergic reaction to an amide local anaesthetic. *Br J Anaesth.* 1981; 53:435–437.

104 McLeskey CH. Allergic reaction to an amide local anaesthetic [letter]. *Br J Anaesth.* 1981; 53:1105–1106.

105 Hall DL, Steen WH, Drummond JW, Byrd WA. Anticoagulants and cataract surgery. *Ophthalmic Surgery* 1988; 19:221–222.

106 McMahan LB. Anticoagulants and cataract surgery. *J Cataract Refract Surg.* 1988; 14:569–571.

107 Stone LS, Kline OR Jr, Sklar C. Intraocular lenses and anticoagulation and antiplatelet therapy. *J Am Intraocul Implant Soc.* 1985; 11:165–168.

108 Gainey SP, Robertson DM, Fay W, Ilstrup D. Ocular surgery on patients receiving long-term warfarin therapy. *Am J Ophthalmol.* 1989; 108:142–146.

109 Robinson GA, Nylander A. Warfarin and cataract extraction. *Br J Ophthalmol.* 1989; 73:702–703.

110 Shuler JD, Paschal JF, Holland GN. Antiplatelet therapy and cataract surgery. *J Cataract Refract Surg.* 1992; 18:567–571.

15

A Vision of the Future

Prof Chris Dodds

Introduction

The changes we shall face in the next fifty years or more of this century will encompass all aspects of ophthalmic anaesthesia and surgery. This is a personal expectation of what will be routine by 2020, and how our practice will have evolved. I have written this as a retrospective view of these changes and I have assumed that the development of medical database access through the Internet and other media has not resulted in the decline of professional medical practice.

It is convenient to use the age of the patients as a guide through these changes in practice.

Intrauterine Care

Developments in four-dimensional ultrasound and colour Doppler imaging ensure that many of the congenital diseases of the eye, orbit and upper face are identified long before 20 weeks of gestation. Developmental problems with the optic vesicles and optic stalk are confirmed at the 3–4 week stage, and disorders of the optic cup by the 5th week. Lens differentiation and normal retinal growth is confirmed. During the following few weeks the normality of the vitreous, choroid and optic blood vessels are reviewed. Where there are indications from these images, confirmed by the routine preimplantation, genome selection assay, corrective surgery is indicated. Fine fibre-optic laser scalpels and tissue adhesives have made such intrauterine surgery safe and effective.

The anaesthetic care of the maternal/foetal complex has been refined to avoid changes in placental function and the teratogenetic effects of the older anaesthetic agents. Combined spinal/epidural techniques are still used in peripheral centres, but increasingly direct spinal cord neuro-modulation preventing c- and aδ-fibres activity from entering ascending pathways or developing local hyperactivity is being used. (The implantation of nano-stimulators by skilled anaesthetists immediately after

conception or more often by guided embryo-selection surgery (GUESS), has revolutionised the provision of anaesthesia during the entire duration of the pregnancy.)

Early Childhood

The elimination of much of the complex oculoplastic paediatric surgery secondary
to congenital disease has limited this field to strabismus and cosmetic surgery.
Adjustable sutures have been replaced by another nano-device, the collagen pulley.
The computer interface linked to the optic cortex continuously monitors binocular
function and uses a feedback loop to lengthen or shorten the pulley almost instanta-
neously. The secondary activation of either lytic or depositional enzymes to modify
the muscle insertions has proved very reliable and effective. The anaesthetic challenges in providing a stable eye, with no blood loss at all, have been overcome by
sleep induction and maintenance techniques (see below). The optic cortex sensor
array is simply injected into the occipital galeal space during the early stages of the
procedure, and fine-tuned by visual evoked potentials.

The concerns of anaesthetists about disorders such as malignant hyperpyrexia or
the muscular dystrophies have long been laid to rest. (They remain on the training
curriculum in the history section.)

However, some cosmetic procedures are becoming more popular as parents strive
to enhance the genetic potential of their children by copying proven facial stereo-
types for success within their chosen field of vocation. Iris re-colouration and orbital
reconfiguration are now routine.

Adulthood

The pattern of ophthalmic practice in caring for adult patients has developed into
social aspects and the residual effects of disease processes that were too far advanced
to respond to current gene therapy.

Social Aspects

The growth in implantable 'head-up' displays for all aspects of social and working
practices has evolved as one of the greatest elements of current practice. The early
primitive displays of an overlay of street maps or of directions to social gatherings
have been replaced by total immersion displays. Social restructuring, necessitated by
the overwhelming growth in population, has been made possible by the interactive
immersion technique of World Objectivity Realism and Culture (WORC). The ability to see and hear as if in an office or hospital has reduced the isolation felt by the
many workers based at home.

The sub-surface corneal surgery required for this has been dependent on the discovery of topical drugs that preserve the endothelial architecture of the cornea whilst
allowing the optic relay grids to accurately project on to the retina. The planned sub-
retinal/optic nerve devices have failed to deliver to date.

Age-related Aspects

Cataract surgery has been revolutionised by the vortex aspiration techniques. Once the technology to create minute, but totally circular capsular entry sites had been perfected it was only a matter of time before cataract surgery for the majority of patients became a 'high-street' procedure. The introduction of dual-phase viscous lens materials was the next advance that allowed titration of implant volume to visual acuity immediately after cataract removal. The malleable nature of the materials returned accommodation to juvenile levels.

Glaucoma care has been improved by implantable nano-pumps that maintain anterior pressure at precisely defined levels. These are inserted under topical anaesthesia and are remotely adjustable from the ophthalmologist's office.

Trauma

The benefits of whole organ tissue culture from cloned material combined with the neuronal regeneration therapy has limited visual loss following trauma to only a few weeks in the majority of cases. The procedures that have been developed to repair or re-implant entire globes are still evolving and provide both surgical and anaesthetic challenges.

Anaesthetic Advances

Anaesthetic Agents

Lipid-based sleep-inducing agents were discovered in the late years of the last century and have been developed into specific agents capable of accurately producing stages 1–4 of NREM sleep. The current lipid induction and maintenance agents have proved to be safe and appear to lack the problems with the hippocampal atrophy seen with the earlier agents. Transcutaneous absorption is one of the key advantages of these agents, and simple massage of the anaesthetic into a vessel rich area is effective within 5 or 10 minutes. Rapid onset of action can still be achieved intravenously where there are clinical indications.

The addition of muscle relaxation by REM-like nucleus tractus solitarius stimulation has completely altered the approach to patient care during surgery. The unbelievable toxicity of the neuronal poisons such as the volatile or intravenous anaesthetic agents is now in the past, and patients are assured of going to sleep and waking on demand as a routine. The degree of hypnosis is determined in advance and the required dosage of lipid is simply massaged into the patient about half an hour prior to transfer to theatre. Reversal is just as straightforward with the adenosine stimulating agents being nasally administered from specially designed filter machines, not dissimilar to the old-fashioned coffee machines.

Airway protection is achieved by the use of the glycine antagonist lozenge developed almost by serendipity in response to the snoring society's drive to harmonise the proximity of the elderly social groupings necessary to meet the demands of a tight-knit ageing society. The strychnine analogues have now become routine medication both in hospital practice and at home.

Anaesthetic Equipment

The Computer Interface for the Anaesthetist (CIA) has developed almost as quickly as the surgical equivalent, and the majority of anaesthetics are now delivered under anaesthetic supervision by remote devices. Monitoring is both real time and predictive. The expertise of the anaesthetist is enhanced by prompts from the CIA about developing trends in the patient physiological status, and there is direct access to the senior supervisors within the department and worldwide to help identify and manage unusual changes.

Minimal flow anaesthesia is routine, the oxygen delivery being constantly adjusted to the metabolic activity of the patient's individual organ systems whilst specific vaso-active agents ensure matching of perfusion to demand. Compact ventilation and monitoring systems are now the size of the small face masks used twenty years ago, or are integrated into laryngeal airways. Telemetry ensures that the anaesthetist is always fully informed of the patient's condition. The entire anaesthetic event is stored by the hospital record system with the contemporary surgical and nursing images, and is available for integration into the training simulators if an educational or technical aspect is present that will be of benefit to trainees.

Hypnosis is usually by induced 'physiological' sleep and its modulation, but volatile agents are still used in some cases. Careful assessment of their respiratory function remains essential to ensure a safe recovery. Intravenous anaesthesia remains the mainstay for rapid induction in emergency situations but is being less frequently used for routine anaesthesia. For most of the major ophthalmic procedures avoidance of any suppression of the optic pathways remains important because of the intra-operative surgical evaluation of function. Direct needle-, or cannula-based anaesthesia in the orbit has been avoided for many years, partly for safety reasons but largely because of the new and more potent topical anaesthetic agents. These can be programmed for deep penetration into the orbital fat where they can continue to deliver anaesthetic concentrations for predetermined durations from a few minutes to several days.

Training

Training and skills evaluation are all simulation-based and anaesthetic trainees will have logged their hours on all aspects of care. The limitation imposed in previous generations by the haphazard presentation of clinical cases no longer occurs, and specialist experience can be gained in a controlled and predictable way. There is little direct clinical access for the first few years of training, and only the most experienced are eligible to visit outlying units. Ophthalmic anaesthesia training for both general and regional orbital block techniques is completed in the main teaching centres and focuses on techniques on patients of all ages. Special emphasis is placed on the understanding of the impact of anaesthetic technique on the eye, its neuronal pathways, and the neuromuscular control.

Summary

Anaesthesia for ophthalmic surgery will remain as a very important element in the total care of ophthalmic patients. However, many aspects will have changed beyond recognition over the next twenty years. Some of these changes will be driven by clinical demand (often overwhelming), some will be due to improvements in anaesthetic drugs and equipment, surgical advances, whilst others will be due to 'intelligent' computing advances. We must ensure that we remain at the forefront of these changes, as leaders of change rather than as followers. After all, it will only be a few more years before we will be the patient rather than the anaesthetist.

Index